The Practical Guide to Clinical Research and Publication

The Practical Guide to Clinical Research and Publication

Uzung Yoon

Assistant Professor, Department of Anesthesiology,
Co-Director of Liver Transplantation Anesthesiology,
Thomas Jefferson University Hospital,
Philadelphia, PA, United States

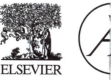

ACADEMIC PRESS

An imprint of Elsevier

Academic Press is an imprint of Elsevier
125 London Wall, London EC2Y 5AS, United Kingdom
525 B Street, Suite 1650, San Diego, CA 92101, United States
50 Hampshire Street, 5th Floor, Cambridge, MA 02139, United States
The Boulevard, Langford Lane, Kidlington, Oxford OX5 1GB, United Kingdom

Notices
Knowledge and best practice in this field are constantly changing. As new research and experience broaden our understanding, changes in research methods, professional practices, or medical treatment may become necessary.

Practitioners and researchers must always rely on their own experience and knowledge in evaluating and using any information, methods, compounds, or experiments described herein. In using such information or methods they should be mindful of their own safety and the safety of others, including parties for whom they have a professional responsibility.

To the fullest extent of the law, neither the Publisher nor the authors, contributors, or editors, assume any liability for any injury and/or damage to persons or property as a matter of products liability, negligence or otherwise, or from any use or operation of any methods, products, instructions, or ideas contained in the material herein.

British Library Cataloguing-in-Publication Data
A catalogue record for this book is available from the British Library

Library of Congress Cataloging-in-Publication Data
A catalog record for this book is available from the Library of Congress

ISBN: 978-0-12-824517-0

For Information on all Academic Press publications
visit our website at https://www.elsevier.com/books-and-journals

Publisher: Stacy Masucci
Acquisitions Editor: Erin Hill-Parks
Editorial Project Manager: Pat Gonzalez
Production Project Manager: Punithavathy Govindaradjane
Cover Designer: Matthew Limbert

Typeset by MPS Limited, Chennai, India

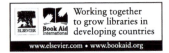

Working together
to grow libraries in
developing countries

www.elsevier.com • www.bookaid.org

Contents

Preface

This book is written for healthcare professionals who want to understand the principles of epidemiology statistics and the application in clinical trials. The content of this textbook is presented in bullet point so that the information is easily accessible to anyone independent of the prior knowledge. The numerous, very clinically oriented examples and drawings are intended to facilitate an understanding and clarify the relationship to clinic and practice.

Many clinical decisions and guidelines are made based on clinical trials. To understand these guidelines and clinical trials and to be able to critically assess them, an understanding of epidemiology and statistics is of particular importance. Busy healthcare practitioners directly involved in patient care can use this book to orient themselves quickly and to gain an overview of epidemiology and statistics and clinical trials.

Apart from this, the book will serve as a guide for the healthcare professionals to design, conduct, and publish their own studies.

Uzung Yoon
Assistant Professor, Department of Anesthesiology,
Co-Director of Liver Transplantation Anesthesiology,
Thomas Jefferson University Hospital, Philadelphia,
PA, United States

Acknowledgment

I would like to acknowledge the reviewers:

Athanasios Magkidis, MD	Department of Radiology, Klinikum Bielefeld Mitte, Bielefeld, Germany
Dejan List, MD	Pediatrics, Dr. med. Dejan List, Wittenberg, Germany
Mau-Thek Eddy, MD	Vice Chairman, Department of Ophthalmology, University Medical Center Hamburg-Eppendorf, Hamburg, Germany
Monika Theis, MD	Department of Anesthesiology, Red Cross Hospital, Bremen, Germany
Philipp Jungebluth, MD	Orthopedics, Sander-Beuermann, Hannover, Germany
Sebastian Witt, MD	Family and Palliative Medicine, Family Medicine at the Theater, Braunschweig, Germany
Susanne Moller, MD	Region Hannover, Team Veterinary Medicine Authority, Hannover, Germany
Kirsi Jonassen, MD	Hannover, Germany
Zizung Yoon, PhD	Institute of Airospace Engineering, Technische Universität Berlin, Berlin, Germany
Lai Lai Kwok, DO	Columbia University, New York, NY, United States
Karsten Knobloch, MD, PhD	Professor, Plastic Hand and Reconstructive Surgery, Hannover Medical School, Hannover, Germany
Linh Ngyuen, MS	Sidney Kimmel Medical College, Thomas Jefferson University Hospital, Philadelphia, PA, United States
Chuck Ngyuen, MD	Department of Anesthesiology, Riverside University Health system, Moreno Valley, CA, United States
Paul Del Prato, MS	Sidney Kimmel Medical College, Thomas Jefferson University Hospital, Philadelphia, PA, United States

Chapter 1

Introduction

Chapter outline

Clinical research in medicine

In medicine, "basic research" or "basic science" involves research and laboratory studies that provide the foundation for clinical research. Research increases our understanding of normal human biology and diseases, and ultimately helps us to discover and develop new treatments or technologies to improve health. About 60% of the NIH budget is allocated for basic research, and most of the basic research funds go to PhD scientists.

Translational research is the process of applying discoveries generated during laboratory research and in preclinical studies to the development of trials and studies in humans. Translational research is specifically designed to transfer findings from laboratory and preclinical research to practice settings and communities, where the findings can improve health outcomes.

Clinical research is the study of health and disease in human subjects (or materials of human origin, such as tissues, specimens, and cognitive phenomena) that directly impacts the patient's health outcome. It uses clinical trials and epidemiological methods to synthesize evidence, to evaluate preventive, therapeutic and diagnostic measurers and to treat illnesses. It is also used in order to study and test new medical equipment, medical procedures, and diagnostic tests. Clinical research describes many different elements of scientific investigation and helps to translate basic research into clinically relevant information to ultimately improve patient care.

The main components of clinical research are epidemiology, statistics, and clinical trials. Epidemiology is the study (scientific, systematic, and data-driven) of the distribution (frequency, pattern) and determinants (causes, risk factors) of health-related states and events (not just diseases) in specified populations (neighborhood, school, city, state, country, global).[i] It is a fundament of medical science and it helps to understand the principles of the methodology in clinical research. Modern epidemiology heavily emphasizes statistics, computer science, genetics, genomics, and bioinformatics. The role of clinical epidemiology is, by way of clinical research, to provide clinicians

The Practical Guide to Clinical Research and Publication.
DOI: https://doi.org/10.1016/B978-0-12-824517-0.00005-8
1

with the information to make decisions that are most appropriate in the best interest of their patients. The information is derived from scientific, evidence-based clinical research and systematic, data-driven analysis.

Statistics refers to both quantitative data, and the classification of such data in accordance with probability theory and the application to them of methods such as hypothesis testing. Medical statistics include both empirical data and estimates related to health, such as mortality, morbidity, risk factors, health service coverage, and health systems.

Clinical trials are experiments or observations done in clinical research. Such research studies on human participants are designed to answer specific questions about biomedical or procedural interventions, including new treatments (such as vaccines, drugs, surgical procedures, and medical devices) and known interventions that warrant further study and comparison. Depending on the product type and development stage, clinical trials can vary in size and cost, and they can involve a single research center or multiple centers, in one country or in multiple countries. The number of new pharmaceuticals, biologics, medical devices, and healthcare services are rapidly expanding and so are clinical trials. The data generated from clinical trials is used to calculate survival information, therapeutic success rates, safety, and efficacy. It is also the fundament for evidence-based medicine, medical guideline development or health policy decision makings.

The decisions made in clinical practice are associated with some uncertainties. This is because medical-biological processes are governed not only by the law of nature but also random factors. Therefore, it is possible to estimate medical-biological processes, but not to calculate their exact value. Epidemiology and statistics are primarily used to first derive a general statement that then forms the theoretical basis for clinical practices. Clinical trials are the foundation of evidence-based medicine. Every day more than 5000 new studies are published in electronic databases. Thus, the number of studies and the information gain is enormous.

In order to interpret the data, and critically assess these clinical trials, one must possess an understanding of the basic principles in conducting a clinical trials, epidemiology, and statistics. This is important in order to understand the fundaments in clinical research for advancing medical knowledge and ultimately improving patient care, whether it being a physician, researcher, or data scientist.

Endnote

i. Dicker R. Principles of epidemiology in public health practice. 3rd ed. CDC; 2006.

Chapter 2

Evidence-based medicine

Chapter outline

Evidence-based medicine

Evidence-based medicine

- In evidence-based medicine (EBM), medical decisions are made on the basis of proven efficacy.
- The efficacy is determined using statistical methods and based on clinical trials (e.g., randomized controlled trials, cohort studies, and case-control studies).
- The term was introduced in the early 1990s by Gordon Guyatt and David Sackett at McMaster University, Hamilton, Canada.

Original quote[i]

The conscientious, explicit and judicious use of current best evidence in making decisions about the care of the individual patient. It means integrating individual clinical expertise with the best available external clinical evidence from systematic research.

David Sackett

- EBM is an approach to medical practice that aims to optimize decision-making by emphasizing the use of the best available evidence from well-designed and well-conducted research.
- Evidence alone does not affect the clinical decision making process. The full combination of the three components; doctor, patient, and evidence, creates "EBM."
- EBM requires education of the clinician in efficient literature-searching, and the application of formal rules of evidence in evaluating the clinical literature.

The Practical Guide to Clinical Research and Publication.
DOI: https://doi.org/10.1016/B978-0-12-824517-0.00012-5

- The practice of EBM is a process of lifelong, self-directed, problem-based learning. Caring for a patient creates the need for clinically important information about diagnosis, prognosis, therapy, and other clinical and health care issues.
- **Doctor**: individual's clinical experience.
- **Patient**: individual's medical problem, patient preference, and patient's will.
- **Evidence**: Best available evidence generated from scientific studies.

Components of EBM (Fig. 2.1).

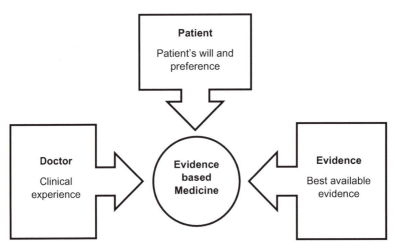

FIGURE 2.1 Components of evidence-based medicine. *Modified after Haynes RB, Devereaux PJ, Guyatt GH. Clinical expertise in the era of evidence-based medicine and patient choice. ACP J Club 2002;136:A11−A14.*

Evidence-based medicine
- Evidence should not be selected based on financial influence or publishing platform (journal, library).
- Literature must be transparent.
  - What previous theoretical knowledge was available?
  - What was the hypothesis, primary and secondary outcome?
  - What method and analytical method were used?
  - Were there any factors that might have an impact on the study (e.g., funding)?
- Timely access to literature must be possible.

Quote:

Essential for evidence-based medicine is the structured and systematic approach with which the most transparent, timely, and undistorted consideration of study results is to be achieved.

Cochrane collaboration[ii]

Methods of EBM in the clinical setting (Fig. 2.2)

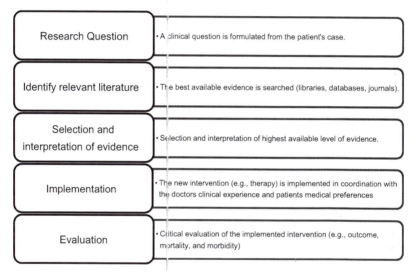

Research Question
• A clinical question is formulated from the patient's case.

Identify relevant literature
• The best available evidence is searched (libraries, databases, journals).

Selection and interpretation of evidence
• Selection and interpretation of highest available level of evidence.

Implementation
• The new intervention (e.g., therapy) is implemented in coordination with the doctors clinical experience and patients medical preferences

Evaluation
• Critical evaluation of the implemented intervention (e.g., outcome, mortality, and morbidity)

FIGURE 2.2   Methods of evidence-based medicine.

Disadvantages of EBM

- Evidence always depends on the viewer's perspective. Therefore, there is no clear evidence.
- The dissemination of research is a very selective process, which creates inevitable research gaps.
    - Not all research is published.
    - Journals selectively choose which research to publish.
    - The evidence (clinical studies) is not always freely accessible.
    - Research follows a certain trend (profitable medication, popular illness [e.g., coronavirus]).
    - Rare diseases are less studied.

- Poor quality studies misrepresent the evidence.
  - Numerous studies with poor study design are published.
  - Funding can influence the study results.
  - There are counterfeit, plagiarized, and duplicated research that is getting published.
- EBM is expensive and slow.
- EBM can influence health care expenditure (waste or reserve).
- The economics of EBM as a system have not been proven.

David Sackett, Gordon Guyatt
    Canadian physician and one of the pioneers of evidence-based medicine at McMaster University in Hamilton (Ontario). David Sackett founded the first university department for clinical epidemiology in 1967.

Science-based medicine

The concept of EBM has been used widely in clinical practice. However, the evidence utilized in EBM is not always generated from scientific studies. The lack of scientific background and scientific explanation of findings in clinical research creates false evidence that is transferred into clinical practice. This problem arises because the goal of biomedical research focuses on finding associations, correlations, risks, benefits, and outcomes based on statistical analysis regardless of the scientific explanation of an association. Often the science aspect is secondary or not evaluated at all. Another problem is the lack of process control for biomedical research. Clinical research and medical practice is very much dependent on culture, politics, economy, funding, and other characteristics of human society.

In general, clinical research conducted with inferior science background lacks reproducibility. This is because the study results are population- and environment-dependent and do not follow a physical or physiological law.

In science-based medicine (SBM) biomedical, physiological, and physical laws do not change regardless of the population or the environment.

Science-based medicine

- A clinical trial should be grounded in scientific plausibility.
- Science is defined as "the intellectual and practical activity encompassing the systematic study of the structure and behavior of the physical and natural laws or world through observation and experiment."
- Science exists as an interdependent network of theories, knowledge, physiology, and laws.
- Science discovers the laws of nature blindly, purposelessly, and without regard to its potential human use.

- Medicine is the application of science to the treatment of illnesses.
- SBM evaluates scientific reasoning, and its plausibility in medical practice.
- SBM endorses EBM's premises and principles, but it also regards it as incomplete.
- EBM's focus on clinical trial results has utility but fails to properly deal with medical modalities that lie outside of the scientific paradigm, or that have scientific plausibility ranging from very little to nonexistent.
- Reproduction of "landmark −studies" is often not possible due to lack of science.

Examples of clinical research that are not science based and the impact.

Example 1

Estimated blood loss (EBL) as an outcome measure that is not based on scientific plausibility.

Evaluating EBL for a specific surgical procedure is a common clinical research question.

The EBL is often calculated based on visual estimation.

- *0−200 mL: mild*
- *200−500 mL: moderate*
- *500−1000 mL: severe*

However, the visual estimation of EBL has 80% variability among estimators. Considering flipping a coin has only 50% variability, the visual estimation of EBL is less reliable and is not grounded in scientific plausibility.

- *Assuming there is no lysis of red blood cells, the biomedical, physiological, and physical laws indicate that a red blood cell mass always remains the same.*
- *Dilutional anemia during surgery and loss of red blood cells on the surgical field is a redistribution of red blood cells, but the total mass remains constant.*
- *The initial red blood cell mass of the patient should be equal to the postsurgical red blood cell mass of the patient plus the red blood cell mass at the surgical field (e.g., sponges, suction canister, and drapes).*
- *Therefore, the scientific approach to calculate EBL would be to measure the initial red blood cell mass of the patient and the postsurgical red blood cell mass of the patient and to calculate the difference.*
- *This is obviously clinically not possible, and therefore a scientific estimation of EBL remains a challenge.*
- *Several methods for EBL estimation have been described (e.g., gravimetric method, colorimetric method, and radioactive tracer injection) but none of them are able to accurately measure EBL and be used in daily clinical research.*

- *Therefore, the question should arise: "should we really need to use EBL as an outcome measure?" If a surgical patient has adequate cardiac output, tissue perfusion, and oxygen delivery to vital organs, the amount of EBL may not affect patient outcome. The scientific plausibility is that the EBL-related decrease in cardiac output and oxygen delivery leads to tissue hypoperfusion and adverse outcome.*

Example 2

Impact of research that is not based on scientific plausibility in the clinical setting.

Aprotinin is an antifibrinolytic medication and was used for many years to limit blood loss for patients undergoing surgical treatment for ST-elevation myocardial infarction. This approach appears counterintuitive since antifibrinolytic medication will inhibit a blood clot from dissolving and can worsen myocardial infarction.

However numerous studies had focused on blood loss as the primary outcome measure instead of the scientific interaction of aprotinin and blood coagulation and concluded that aprotinin decreased blood loss.

Mangano et al.[iii] published a paper in 2006 that stated: "Use of aprotinin in the latter group was associated with a 55% increase in the risk of myocardial infarction or heart failure (P < .001) and a 181% increase in the risk of stroke or encephalopathy (P = .001). The association between aprotinin and serious end-organ damage indicates that continued use is not prudent."

- *After this study was published aprotinin was removed from the market.*
- *For decades patient were treated with aprotinin and were exposed to a higher risk of stroke and myocardial infarction. This example clearly demonstrates the impact of nonscientific based clinical research, generating false evidence and leading to harm in patient care.*

Biomedical literature databases (Table 2.1)

TABLE 2.1 List of biomedical databases.

Database	Website
PUBMED (MEDLINE)	http://www.pubmed.com
EMBASE	http://www.embase.com
NLM (National Library of Medicine)	http://www.nlm.nih.gov/
NCBI (National Center for Biotechnology Information)	http://www.ncbi.nlm.nih.gov/
Cochrane	http://www.cochrane.org
Google Scholar	https://scholar.google.com/
Scopus	https://www.scopus.com/

The largest medical databases are PubMed and EMBASE.

PubMed

- PUBMED (http://www.pubmed.gov) is owned by the United States National Library of Medicine National Institutes of Health
- It includes more than 20 million publications.
- PUBMED is the largest component of the United States National Library of Medicine's® (NLM) literature database and MEDLINE (Medical Literature Analysis and Retrieval System Online).
- 2000–4000 new publications are published every week.

National Library of Medicine (NLM)

- NLM has nearly 12 million books, journals, manuscripts, audiovisuals, and other forms of medical information, making it the largest health-science library in the world.
- The most frequently consulted online scientific medical resource in the world is MEDLINE®/PubMed®, a publicly available database of over 18 million journal citations from 1948 to the present.

MEDLINE

- MEDLINE is the United States National Library of Medicine's® (NLM) premier bibliographic database that contains over 19 million references to journal articles in life sciences with a concentration on biomedicine.
- A distinctive feature of MEDLINE is that the records are indexed with NLM Medical Subject Headings (MeSH®).
- MEDLINE is the primary component of PubMed®, part of the Entrez series of databases provided by the NLM National Center for Biotechnology Information (NCBI).
- Time coverage: generally 1946 to the present, with some older material.

EMBASE

- Contains more than 24 million indexed documents and more than 7600 journals.
- More journals (8500) than MEDLINE
- Catalog of conference abstracts
- More coverage of non-English content
- Journal coverage from 1947 to the present
- Over 1.5 million records added yearly, with an average of over 6000 each day
- All MEDLINE records produced by the NLM are included, as well over 5 million records not covered on MEDLINE (Fig. 2.3).

Cochrane Library

- The Cochrane Library is a collection of databases in medicine.
- At its core is the collection cochrane database of systematic reviews (CDSR), a database of systematic reviews and *meta*-analyses which summarize and interpret the results of medical research. It is the leading journal and database for systematic reviews in health care.

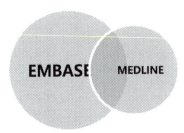

FIGURE 2.3 Diagram comparing EMBASE and MEDLINE (PubMed) database. *Wilkins T, Gillies RA, Davies K. EMBASE vs MEDLINE for family medicine searches: can MEDLINE searches find the forest or a tree? Can Fam Physician 2005;51:848−9.*

- Cochrane produces high-quality, relevant, up-to-date systematic reviews and other synthesized research evidence to inform health decision making.
- There are now over 7500 cochrane systematic reviews which we publish in the cochrane library.

Scopus
- Scopus, launched in November 2004, is the largest abstract and citation database containing both peer-reviewed research literature and quality web sources.
- It contains over 19,000 titles from more than 5000 international publishers.
- It contains 46 million records, 70% with abstracts and over 4.6 million conference papers.

Google Scholar
- Released in November 2004, the google scholar index includes most peer-reviewed online journals of Europe and America's largest scholarly publishers, plus scholarly books other nonpeer reviewed journals.
- Google Scholar is a freely accessible web search engine that indexes the full text of scholarly literature.

Endnotes

i. Sackett DL, Rosenberg WM, Gray JA, Haynes RB, Richardson WS. Evidence based medicine: what it is and what it isn't. BMJ 1996;312:71−2.
ii. The cochrane collaboration—http://www.cochrane.org
iii. Mangano DT, Tudor IC, Dietzel C; Multicenter Study of Perioperative Ischemia Research Group; Ischemia Research and Education Foundation. The risk associated with aprotinin in cardiac surgery. N Engl J Med. 2006 26;354:353−65.

Chapter 3

Epidemiology

Chapter outline

Definition and classification

Definition of epidemiology

Epidemiology is the science and study of the cause, consequence, spread, and prevention of a disease affecting an individual or a larger population.

Other definitions
- The study of the distribution and determinants of health-related states or events in specified populations and the application of this study to control health problems (Last 2001).[i]
- The study of the distribution and determinants of disease frequency in human populations (MacMahon, 1970).[ii]
- The study of the distribution of health-related states and events in populations (Rothman et al., 2008).[iii]

Targets of epidemiology are to
- Validate and to precisely estimate the frequency of occurrence of health conditions.
- Validate and to precisely estimate the effect of exposure in order to identify possible causes for the development of a disease.
- Describe and explain the distribution of health and illness within and between populations.
- Identify risk factors.
- Explain the etiology and prognosis of diseases.
- Investigate the effectiveness of interventions and health measures.

The Practical Guide to Clinical Research and Publication.
DOI: https://doi.org/10.1016/B978-0-12-824517-0 00011-3

- Give recommendations on clinical care and policy measures.

Shortcoming of epidemiology
- The basic strategy of epidemiology is to compare groups of people.
- Only fair comparisons can give reliable estimates of associations.

Classification

Descriptive epidemiology
- Descriptive epidemiology deals with the description of the frequency of certain diseases or health disorders and their distribution in the population.
- Descriptive epidemiology is a prerequisite for analytical epidemiology.

Analytical epidemiology
- Analytical epidemiology tries to obtain clues to causal factors through hypothesis testing.
- Examines relationships between exposure and outcome using statistical calculations.
- Judges whether an association is valid and if there is causality.
- A reliable descriptive epidemiology is a prerequisite for analytical epidemiology.

Epidemiological methods

Traditional census
- The direct questioning of the entire population by means of questionnaires or interviews.

Register census
- Obtains the required information from existing administrative registers.
- Not a direct questioning of the population.

Rolling census
- Continuous annual data collection by means with a direct survey.
- The scope of the surveys mostly depends on the size of the municipality.

Mixed forms
- Combination of traditional census and data collection through the use of registers.
- Or register censuses is supplemented with a sample from a population.

Micro census
- Households that are selected according to random criteria are interviewed.
- Usually 1% sample of all private households are surveyed.

- Serves for official representative statistics about a defined population and the labor market.

Epidemiological study types

Epidemiological methods are used to determine the relationship between exposure and risk factors in a disease. Epidemiological studies are classified into observational studies (ecological studies, cross-sectional study, cohort study, and case-control study) and intervention studies (randomized controlled study, controlled clinical study, and community intervention study) (Fig. 3.1).

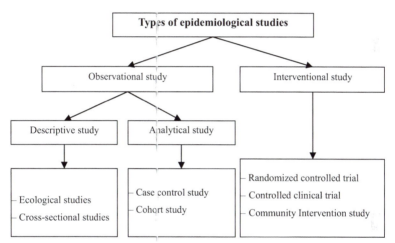

FIGURE 3.1   Types of epidemiological studies.

Association and causality

Association

- An association describes a pure relationship between two or more events without causality.

Causality

- A causality describes the relationship between cause and effect with the idea that "every event (outcome) is caused by a previous event (exposure)"

Example

Smoking causes lung cancer.

Criteria for assessing the causality of an association

Sir Austin Bradford Hill described eight criteria that can be used in assessing the causality of a discovered association[iv]:

1. Strength
2. Consistency
3. Temporality
4. Dose-response relationship
5. Biological plausibility
6. Reversibility
7. Specificity
8. Coherence

1. Strength of the relationship
   a. The stronger the association between exposure and outcome, the more likely a causal relationship exists.
   b. A strong association reduces the likelihood that an observed effect is caused by confounders.
   c. A weak association can be causal but is more difficult to identify.
   d. Not every causal relationship is based on a strong association.
   e. The strength of the association also depends on other existing causal factors.

2. Relationship consistency
   a. There is strong evidence of causality when different scientists study a different population, using different study methods and still find similar results.

3. Temporal sequence
   a. Exposure must precede the outcome.
   b. Only if the exposure precedes the outcome, it can be causal.
   c. However, not every exposure that precedes an outcome is automatically a cause. (e.g., smoking and liver cancer).

4. Dose-effect relationship
   a. Does the risk of illness increase with increasing exposure?
   b. Problems:
      i. Dose-response relationships can be caused by confounders.
      ii. Dose-impact relationships may not exist if there is a threshold effect.
      iii. Some causal associations show a threshold effect.

5. Biological plausibility
   a. Is there a rational and theoretical basis for the association?
   b. Does the association makes sense?
   c. If there is no described biological plausible mechanism, this could be due to a lack of knowledge.

6. Reversibility
   a. If the frequency of illness is reduced by eliminating the exposure, this strengthens the evidence for a causal relationship.

7. Specificity of the effect
   a. Outcome is predicted by a factor.
   b. Ideally, every factor predicts an outcome.
   c. Sometimes one factor causes multiple outcomes. For example, smoking causes many diseases (COPD, lung cancer, pancreatic carcinoma, etc.).
8. Coherence
   a. Results are in line with existing knowledge.

Further literature

Frérot M, Lefebvre A, Aho S, Callier P, Astruc K, Aho Glélé LS. What is epidemiology? Changing definitions of epidemiology 1978–2017. PLoS One 2018;10 (13):e0208442.

MacMahon B, Pugh TF. Epidemiologic methods. Boston, MA: Little, Brown; 1960; reissued as Epidemiology: Principles and methods. Boston, MA: Little, Brown; 1970. ISBN 0316542593

Last JM. A dictionary of epidemiology. 4th ed. New York; Oxford; Toronto: Oxford University Press; 1988.

Hill, AB. The environment and disease: association or causation? Proc R Soc Med 1965;58(5): 295–300.

Epidemiologic measures

Frequency measures

- Frequency measures are important parameters that give us a first impression about the rate of a disease. These numbers make a comparison among different diseases easier (Table 3.1).

TABLE 3.1 Frequently used measures of mortality.

Measure	Numerator	Denominator	10^n
Crude death rate	Total number of deaths during a given time interval	Mid-interval population	1000 or 100,000
Cause-specific death rate	Number of deaths assigned to a specific cause during a given time interval	Mid-interval population	100,000
Proportionate mortality	Number of deaths assigned to a specific	Total number of deaths from all causes during the same time interval	100 or 1000

(Continued)

TABLE 3.1 (Continued)

Measure	Numerator	Denominator	10^n
	cause during a given time interval		
Death-to-case ratio	Number of deaths assigned to a specific cause during a given time interval	Number of new cases of same disease reported during the same time interval	100
Neonatal mortality rate	Number of deaths among children <28 days of age during a given time interval	Number of live births during the same time interval	1000
Postneonatal mortality rate	Number of deaths among children 28–364 days of age during a given time interval	Number of live births during the same time interval	1000
Infant mortality rate	Number of deaths among children <1 year of age during a given time interval	Number of live births during the same time interval	1000
Maternal mortality rate	Number of deaths assigned to pregnancy-related causes during a given time interval	Number of live births during the same time interval	100,000

Prevalence

Prevalence is the frequency of an illness in a population at a specific point in time. Usually the population size is defined in 10,000 or 100,000 people.

$$\text{Prevalence} = \frac{\text{Number of cases in the population}}{\text{Number of people in the population}}$$

Example 1

On January 1, 2012, in a population of 8000 people, 10 people had diabetes.
   → *Prevalence = 10/8000 = 0.00125*

Example 2

In 2012, in a population of 8000 people, 200 people had diabetes.
   → *Prevalence = 200/8000 = 0.025*
   The prevalence should always be listed in connection with the time of data collection.

Depending on the time period prevalence are defined as:

- **Point prevalence**: prevalence at a certain point in time.
- **Period prevalence**: prevalence in a certain time period.
- **Lifetime prevalence**: prevalence over a lifetime.

Incidence
- The frequency of a new illness.
- The number of newly occurring illnesses within a defined population group for a certain period (e.g., 1 year, 5 years, 10 years).
- In medical literature, the "incidence" often means the incidence rate.

Incidence rate
- Describes the new illness of a certain period of time (usually 100,000) who are exposed to a certain risk. The period is usually defined as 1 year. It can also be specified in months, days, hours, etc.

Example

In 2012, 2000 new diabetes cases were diagnosed in city A. (100,000 residents)
   → Incidence = 2000/100,000 = 0.02 = 2%

Person years
- Special attention should be paid to observation periods in cohort studies and clinical studies that are presented in person-years.

Example

In a city A, the lung cancer risk is 5 times higher than in city B, in relation to 100 people per year.

- ***100 person-years can be:***
  - *100 people observed for 1 year*
  - *50 people observed for 2 years*
  - *10 people observed for 10 years*
  - *5 people observed for 20 years*
  - *1 person observed for 100 years*

Birth rate = Crude birth rate = CBR
- Number of live births per year based on 1000 residents

$$= \frac{\text{Number of live birth per year}}{\text{Total population}} \cdot 1000$$

Fertility rate

$$= \frac{\text{Number of live birth}}{\text{Number of fertile women}} \cdot 1000$$

- Fertile women = women from 15 to 44 years.

Infant mortality
- Number of deaths in children before the age of 1.
- Defined for 1000 live births.

Neonatal mortality
- Number of deaths in children <28 days of age during a given time interval.

Postneonatal mortality
- Number of deaths in children between the second and twelfth month (28−364 days) of life.

Morbidity
- The number/frequency of illnesses of the individuals in a population during a certain time period who have suffered a certain illness.
- Usually based on 10,000 or 100,000 people.

Mortality = death rate (Mortality)
- The number of deaths in a given time period.
- Based on 1000 individuals in a population.
- The period is usually defined as 1 year

$$\textbf{Mortality} = \text{Incidence} \times \text{lethality}$$

$$\text{Crudemortality rate} = \frac{\text{Number of death in a year}}{\text{Total Population}} \cdot 1000$$

- Based on 1000 or 100,0000 individuals

$$\text{Age} - \text{specific mortality rate} = \frac{\text{Number of death in a particular age group}}{\text{Total population in the age group}} \cdot 1000$$

- An age-specific mortality rate is a mortality rate limited to a particular age group.

$$\text{Case} - \text{specific mortality rate} = \frac{\text{Number of death due to a specific reason}}{\text{Total population}} \cdot 1000$$

$$\text{Disease} - \text{specific mortality rate} = \frac{\text{Number of death due to a specific disease}}{\text{Total polulation}} \cdot 1000$$

Lethality
- The ratio of deaths by a certain disease to the number of patients in a given period.

$$\text{Lethality rate} = \frac{\text{Number of death due to a specific disease}}{\text{Number of people affected by a specific disease}}$$

Life expectancy

Normal lifespan
- The average age at which most of the cohort dies.

Average life expectancy
- Years a newborn is expected to live.

Further life expectancy
- Years that a person of a certain age is expected to live.

Probable lifespan
- Age at which half of a certain birth-year is still alive or has already died.

Quality adjusted life years = QALY
- Key figure for evaluating a year of life in relation to health.
- A QALY of 1 means a year in full health, while a QALY of 0 means death.
- If someone is still alive with a disability after a treatment then a value between 0 and 1 is assigned.

Disability adjusted life years = DALY
- DALY = YLD + YLL.
- YLD—*Years of Life lost*: years of life lived with disabilities.
- YLL—*Years lived with Disability*: *Years of* life lost through premature death and disability.

Standardization

Crude rates
- A crude rate is related to a total population.
- It is the number of new cases (or deaths) occurring in a specified population per year.
- Usually, it is expressed as the number of cases per 100,000 individuals (population at risk).
- Comparison between two crude rates can be misleading because populations may differ in characteristics.

Benefits
- Crude rate is easy to calculate.
- It describes the absolute order of magnitude.

Disadvantage
- Comparison of crude rates is difficult because each population has a different age and gender distribution.

Example
Mortality rate- USA 8.3 versus Germany 5.4 versus South Korea 6.7

Standardized rates
- Standardized rates are adjusted rates that consider the differences between populations that influence their crude rate.
- Standardized rates have undergone a statistical transformation to allow the comparison of rates across populations that are different in the distribution of characteristics (e.g., age, sex) that may affect the risk of the disease.
- Standardized rates are statistical measures of any rates in a population.
- It calculates the rates independent from variables in a population.
- It tries to balance out the heterogeneous structures (age, gender, etc.) to enable an equal and fair comparison.

Standardization
- Direct standardization.
- Indirect standardization.
- Age, sex, etc. standardization.

Direct standardization
- Direct standardization is used when the number of events or the mortality rates in each age group within the population, is known.
- The purpose of standardization is to facilitate comparison of rates by removing the effect of composition.
- During the direct standardization study rate (e.g., mortality) of the study population is converted into a standard population.

Example

Comparison before standardization

Country A

Age	Diabetes cases	Population
30–49	100	10,000
50–69	200	4000
> 70	150	1000
Total	450	15,000

$$= \frac{450}{15,000} \bullet 1000$$

$= \rightarrow 30$ *in 1000 people have diabetes*

Country B

Age	Diabetes cases	Population
30–49	60	6000
50–69	200	4000
> 70	750	5000
Total	1010	15,000

$$= \frac{1010}{15000} \bullet 1000$$

→ 67.3 in 1000 people have diabetes
Country B has a higher diabetes rate of 67.3 out of 1000 people than
Country A with only 30 in 1000 people.

Compared after standardization
Predefined standard population

Age	Predefined standard population
30–49	16,000
50–69	8000
> 70	6000

Country A

Age	Diabetes cases	Population	Morbidity rate/1000 people	Predefined standard population	Standardized incidence of diseases
30–49	100	10,000	10	**16,000**	**160**
50–69	200	4000	50	**8000**	**400**
> 70	150	1000	150	**6000**	**900**
Total	450	15,000		**30,000**	**1460**

Country A had a diabetes incidence rate of 1460, after conversion according to the standard population.
Country B

Age	Diabetes cases	Population	Morbidity rate/1000 people	Predefined standard population	Standardized incidence of diseases
30–49	60	6000	10	**16,000**	**160**
50–69	200	4000	50	**8000**	**400**
> 70	750	5000	150	**6000**	**900**
Total	1010	15,000		**30,000**	**1460**

Country B had a diabetes incidence rate of 1460, after conversion according to the standard population.

Country A and Country B have the same diabetes rate of 1460, after conversion according to the standard population.

The reason that the raw data showed a difference between country A and B is due to the higher age population in country B.

Indirect standardization
- Indirect standardization is used when the number of events or the mortality rates in each age group within the population is not known.
- The standard rate (preexisting data) is converted into the study population.

Example

Study A is studying the lung cancer incidence of town A near a factory.

Age	Study population	Lung cancer cases
30–49	10,000	5
50–69	5000	8
> 70	8000	12
Total	15,000	70

Is the lung cancer incidence high or low?
This can be evaluated with indirect standardization.

Age	Studies population	Lung cancer incidence in country A (Preexisting data)	Lung cancer cases after indirect standardization
30–49	10,000	**10**	1
50–69	5000	**20**	0.5
> 70	8000	**30**	0.24
Total	15,000	**100,000**	

Town A lung cancer cases	Country A lung cancer cases after indirect standardization
5	1
8	0.5
12	0.24

Town A has a significantly increased incidence of lung cancer compared to the normal population of country A.

Age standardization
- Commonly used method of standardization besides gender.
- Often used in cancer registries to compare morbidity or mortality rates.
- If there are different age distributions for a study population in two different regions, their mortality or morbidity rates are only comparable to a limited extent.
- After age standardization, data from different years or regions can be compared without the effect of different age distribution.

Standard population = Reference population
- A standard population, often referred to as standard millions, are the age distributions used for age standardizations or to create age-adjusted statistics.
- Common so-called reference populations of age standardization are the Segi world population, European standard populations, and WHO standard population (Table 3.2).[v]

TABLE 3.2 Canadian, European, and world standard population.

Age	European (Scandinavian 1960) std million[1,2]	European (EU-27 plus EFTA 2011–30) std million	World (Segi 1960) std million[1,2]	2000 United States std million	2011 Canadian std population	World (WHO 2000–25) std[2]
00 years	16,000	10,000	24,000	13,818	376,321	17,917
01–04 years	64,000	40,000	96,000	55,317	1,522,743	70,652
05–09 years	70,000	55,000	100,000	72,533	1,810,433	86,870
10–14 years	70,000	55,000	90,000	73,032	1,918,164	85,970
15–19 years	70,000	55,000	90,000	72,169	2,238,952	84,670
20–24 years	70,000	60,000	80,000	66,478	2,354,354	82,171
25–29 years	70,000	60,000	80,000	64,529	2,369,841	79,272
30–34 years	70,000	65,000	60,000	71,044	2,327,955	76,073
35–39 years	70,000	70,000	60,000	80,762	2,273,087	71,475
40–44 years	70,000	70,000	60,000	81,851	2,385,918	65,877
45–49 years	70,000	70,000	60,000	72,118	2,719,909	60,379
50–54 years	70,000	70,000	50,000	62,716	2,691,260	53,681
55–59 years	60,000	65,000	40,000	48,454	2,353,090	45,484
60–64 years	50,000	60,000	40,000	38,793	2,050,443	37,187

(Continued)

TABLE 3.2 (Continued)

Age	European (Scandinavian 1960) std million[1,2]	European (EU-27 plus EFTA 2011–30) std million	World (Segi 1960) std million[1,2]	2000 United States std million	2011 Canadian std population	World (WHO 2000–25) std[2]
65–69 years	40,000	55,000	30,000	34,264	1,532,940	29,590
70–74 years	30,000	50,000	20,000	31,773	1,153,822	22,092
75–79 years	20,000	40,000	10,000	26,999	919,338	15,195
80–84 years	10,000	25,000	5000	17,842	701,140	9097
85 + years	10,000	25,000	5000	15,508	643,070	6348
Total	1,000,000	1,000,000	1,000,000	1,000,000	34,342,780	1,000,000

https://seer.cancer.gov/stdpopulations/stdpop.19ages.html.

Further literature in epidemiology
- Gordis L. Epidemiology. 4th ed. Philadelphia: W.B. Saunders; 2008. ISBN-10: 1416040021
- Last JM. A dictionary of epidemiology. 4th ed. New York, Oxford, Toronto: Oxford University Press; 1988.

Endnotes

i. Last JM, editor. Dictionary of epidemiology. 4th ed. New York: Oxford University Press; 2001. p. 61.

ii. MacMahon B, Pugh TF. Epidemiology: principles and methods. Boston, MA: Little, Brown; 1970. 408 p.

iii. Rothman KJ, Greenland S, Lash TL. Modern epidemiology. Philadelphia, PA: Lippincott Williams & Wilkins; 2008. 776 p.

iv. Howick J, Glasziou P, Aronson JK. The evolution of evidence hierarchies: what can Bradford Hill's guidelines for causation' contribute? J R Soc Med 2009 May;102 (5):186−94.

v. https://seer.cancer.gov/stdpopulations/ 2021; Accessed 01.31.2021.

Chapter 4

Biostatistics

Chapter outline

Fundamentals of statistics

Mean value
- The mean value is the arithmetic mean.
- It is calculated as the quotient of the sum of all observed values divided by the number of observed values.

Median
- The median is the value that is in the middle when all of the values are arranged in ascending order.
- 50% of the values are above and 50% of the values are below the median.

Modal value
- The modal value is the value that appears most often in a set of data (Fig. 4.1).

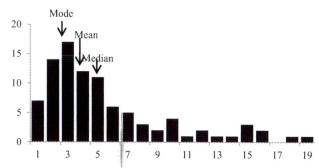

FIGURE 4.1 Mean, median, and modal values.

The Practical Guide to Clinical Research and Publication.
DOI: https://doi.org/10.1016/B978-0-12-824517-0.00002-2

Geometric mean
- The geometric mean is calculated for outliers or for growth rates.
  - 1, 2, 4, 3, 1, 2, 1, 3, 50
  - growth of 5%, 3%, 1%
- The geometric mean never exceeds the arithmetic mean.

Quantile
- A quantile defines a particular part of a data set.
- Quantile defines how many values in a distribution are above or below a certain limit.
- Quintile (fifth), quartile (quarter), median, percentile (hundredth).

Variance
- Variance is a measurement of the spread between numbers in a data set.
- Variance is the expectation of the squared deviation of a random variable from its mean.

Standard deviation
- Standard deviation is a measure of how spread out the numbers are.
- Standard deviation is the square root of the variance.

Example

X axis: height in cm, Y axis: frequency

N	7084
Mean	169.43
Median	169.10
Variance	89.603
Standard deviation	9.466
Minimum	139.4
Maximum	202.0
Percentile	
25	162.5
50	169.1
75	176.1

Graphics in statistics

Histogram (Fig. 4.2 and Fig. 4.3)

- A histogram is a graphical display of continuous sample data using bars of different heights.

Histogramm

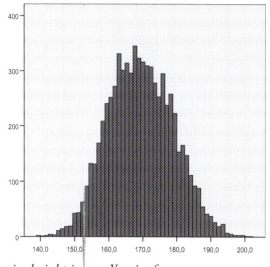

X axis: height in cm, Y axis: frequency

FIGURE 4.2   Histogram and basic statistical values.

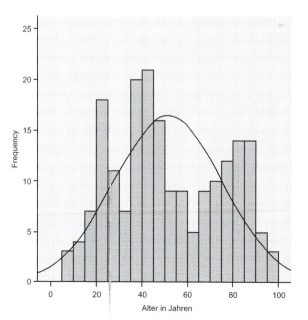

FIGURE 4.3   Histogram.

- A histogram is a graphical display of continuous sample data using bars of different heights.
- It is similar to a bar chart. The difference is that, in a histogram, each bar groups numbers into ranges.
- Taller bars show that more data falls in that range than a shorter bar.

Pros

- Histograms allow viewers to easily compare data.
- The distribution of the variables is easy to recognize.
- The deviation from the ideal distribution can be identified with an overlying Gaussian curve.

Box plot (Fig. 4.4)

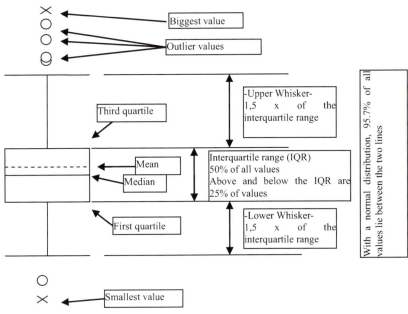

FIGURE 4.4 Box plot.

Pros

- The scattering of the sample values is easily recognizable.
- The box plot provides a lot of information in a single figure.

Scatter plot

- A scatter plot is used to plot data points on a horizontal "X" and a vertical "Y" axis to show how much one variable is affected by the other.

- Dots are used to represent each values for two different numeric variables.
- Scatter plots can provide a quick overview of a large number of variables and observe the relationships between those variables (Fig. 4.5).

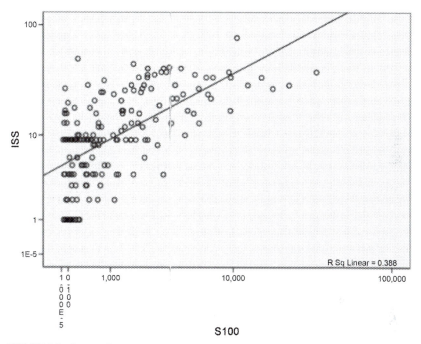

FIGURE 4.5   Scatter plot.

Data distribution

Normal distribution

- Gaussian distribution or bell curve is known as a normal data distribution.
- Mean = median = modal
- In statistics, it is often assumed that the study population has a normal distribution.
- Most measurement techniques and mathematical calculations are based on the assumption of normal distribution (Fig. 4.6).

A bell curve shows the normal distribution of variables according to Carl Friedrich Gauss.

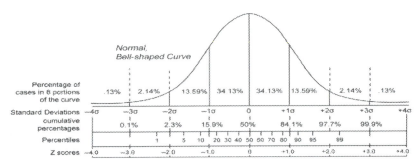

FIGURE 4.6   Gaussian curve.

Left-shifted distribution
- Most of the measured values are shifted to the left.
- Center value > median > modal (Fig. 4.7).

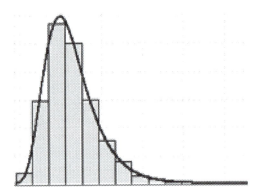

FIGURE 4.7   Left-shifted distribution.

Right-shifted distribution
- Most of the measured values are shifted to the right.
- Mean < median < modal (Fig. 4.8).

Significance value

P-value

Significance test (hypothesis testing)
- For a hypothesis testing, first it is assumed that a treatment or a drug A is not effective.
- If the data collection and statistical analysis shows that "the probability that the drug is not effective is below the significant level," then drug A is considered to be effective.

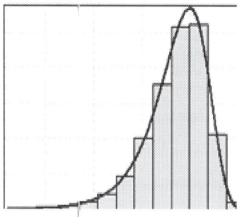

FIGURE 4.8   Right-shifted distribution.

P-value
- The letter p stands for "probability."
- The *P*-value is the probability that the null-hypothesis is true.
- The smaller the *P*-value, the greater the statistical significance (stronger evidence in favor of the alternative hypothesis).
- The *P*-value does not describe the amount of difference. It only indicates that the difference is significant.
- The clinical interpretation of a *P*-value is therefore limited.
- In biomedical statistics and medicine, $P < 0.05$ is considered to be statistically significant.
- The *P*-value > 0.05 only indicates that the null hypothesis cannot be rejected. This does not mean that the null hypothesis is correct. (Missing evidence does not mean that there is no evidence).

Definitions of the *P*-value:
1. The *P*-value is the probability, if the null hypothesis is valid, of finding a value of the test statistic (z) as large or larger than the observed value. Reject the null hypothesis if the *P*-value is less than a predetermined value (< 0.05).
2. The *P*-value is the evidence of the data against the null hypothesis. Reject the null hypothesis if the *P*-value is small.

$P < 0.05$
- $P < 0.05$ is established in medical research as a cutoff value and interpreted that there is a significant effect.

- It indicates that there is less than a 5% probability that the effect of the alternative hypothesis is caused by a random factor.
- In other words, the expected effect is explained in over 95% by the treatment or for example, medication and not by random factors.
- The null hypothesis should be rejected in this case.
  H0: The drug A lowers blood pressure.
  H1: The drug A does not lower blood pressure.
  P = 0.03 (significant)

*Interpretation: Drug A **lowers** the blood pressure with the significance level of P = 0.03.*

  H0: The drug B lowers blood pressure.
  H1: The drug B does not lower blood pressure.
  P = 0.17 (not significant)

*Interpretation: Drug B does **not lower** the blood pressure with the significance level of P = 0.17.*

> **Clinical interpretation of the *P*-value in medicine**
> If the *P*-value is below 0.05 (*P* < 0.05), the desired effect is statistically significant and we accept the alternative hypothesis.

P > 0.05
- *If the P-value is > 0.05 it is interpreted as a nonsignificant effect.*
- *The null-hypothesis cannot be rejected.*
- *However, P > 0.05 does not mean that there is no difference in the effect of treatment.*
- *A clear conclusion is not possible.*

Example

  Group A: The drug lowers mortality by 10%.
  Group B: The drug lowers mortality by 12%.
  P = 0.25 (not significant)

  Correct conclusion:
  There is no statistically significant difference in the mortality reduction between group A and group B.
  Incorrect conclusion:
  The mortality reduction in group A and group B is the same.

Limitation of a significance test
- A decision is only made between $P < 0.05$ or $P > 0.05$.

- Values such as 0.049 (4.9%) or 0.051 (5.1%) that are almost identical are differentiated according to "either or" principle into "significant" and "not significant."
- The statistical significance depends on the number of cases.
- A sufficiently large number of cases can make any small difference in the study significant.
- The null hypothesis is almost never really true.
- A statistical significance does not give any information regarding clinical relevance, significance, or effect.
- An "insignificant" result does not mean that there is no difference.
- Problem of "multiple testing": Some clinical trials perform repeated statistical testing until a statistical significance is found. If enough random testing is performed, the likelihood to find a significant result increases.
- P-value is often in the middle ground of the evaluation and is over-interpreted.
- Studies with insignificant P-values are published less frequently.
- A lower P-value ($P < 0.0001$) shows no greater difference than a higher P-value ($P < 0.05$).
- Interpretations such as "strong/very strong/high/highly significant" are not appropriate.

Confidence interval (Fig. 4.9)

Scattering of measurement errors

- 68.27% of all measured values can be found in the interval of deviation $\pm 1\ \sigma$ from the mean.
- 95.45% of all measured values can be found in the interval of deviation $\pm 2\ \sigma$ from the mean.

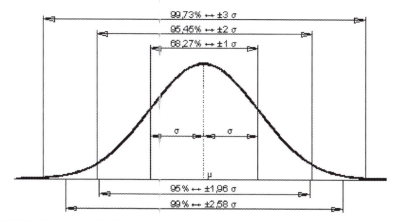

FIGURE 4.9   Normal distribution and standard deviation.

- 99.73% of all measured values can be found in the interval of the deviation $\pm 3\,\sigma$ from the mean.

Deviations from the mean

Conversely, for a given probability, the maximum deviations from the mean are:

- 50% of all measurements have a deviation of 0.675 σ from the mean.
- 90% of all measurements have a deviation of 1.645 σ from the mean.
- 95% of all measurements have a deviation of 1.960 σ from the mean.
- 99% of all measurements have a deviation of 2.575 σ from the mean.

Confidence interval

- The confidence interval indicates the "reliability" of a measurement or estimate.
- The confidence interval is an area that is very likely to cover the real parameter (precision).
- It is an interval estimate of a population parameter.
- A confidence interval level should be defined first (usually 95% or 99%).
- In medicine, a 95% confidence interval is most commonly used.
- If the significance level is α, the confidence level is $1-\alpha$ ($\alpha = 0.05$, confidence level $= 1-\alpha = 0.95 = 95\%$).
- The advantage of the confidence interval over a P-value is the possible clinical interpretation of the strength of the effect.
- A confidence interval depends on sample size.
- A 99% confidence interval is wider than a 95% confidence interval.
- The wider the confidence interval, the less precise the estimated value (Table 4.1; Fig. 4.10).

95% confidence interval

- A 95% confidence is the probability that the value of a randomly selected sample is within the predefined confidence interval range.
- A 95% confidence interval is a range of values, that contains with a 95% certainty the true mean of the population.

TABLE 4.1 Confidence interval and standard score (z).

Confidence interval (%)	Standard score (z)
50	0.67
68	1.00
90	1.64
95	1.96
99	2.58

One sided confidence interval

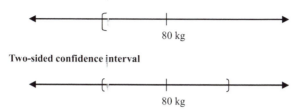

80 kg

Two-sided confidence interval

80 kg

FIGURE 4.10   One sided and two-sided confidence interval.

A significant confidence interval of $\alpha = 0.05$ ($P = 0.05$) exists when:
- Calculating the differences between two mean values (*T*-test): the 95% confidence interval does not include the 0.
- Calculating odds ratio/relative risk (chi-square test): the 95% confidence interval does not include 1 (Fig. 4.11).

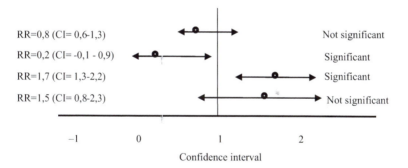

FIGURE 4.11   Example of significant and nonsignificant confidence intervals.

How to clinically interpret a confidence interval:

Example 1

Statistical analysis on a blood pressure difference between two mean values.

Group A: 160 mmHg, Group B: 150 mmHg, P < .05, CI = 5.9−10.3

Interpretation:
P-value <.05 only indicates that there is a significant difference.
Confidence interval indicates that the effect lies with 95% probability in the range of 5.9−10.3 mmHg.

Confidence interval of a proportion
- *(1−α) confidence interval*

$$\text{Confidence interval} = p \pm z1 - \alpha/2\sqrt{p(1-p)/n}$$

z = constant (95% CI: z = 1.96, 99% CI: z = 2.58), p = frequency/proportion, n = number of cases

- *Clopper Pearson confidence interval.*
- *Wilson score interval.*

Confident interval for an average
- *(1−α) confidence interval*

$$\text{Confidence interval} = X \pm z_{1-\alpha/2}\frac{s}{\sqrt{n}}$$

95% confidence interval

$$\text{CI} = X \pm z\frac{s}{\sqrt{n}}$$

$$= \text{Mean} \pm \text{Constant}\frac{\text{Standard deviation}}{\sqrt{\text{number of cases}}}$$

X is the mean, z is the constant (95% CI: $z = 1.96$, 99% CI: $z = 2.58$), s is the standard deviation, n is the number of cases.

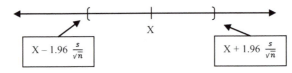

Example

The body weight of 100 patients was measured. The average patient weight was 80 kg.
   Standard deviation is 20 kg.

N = 100
Average weight = 80 kg
Standard deviation = 20 kg

Lower confidence interval	Upper confidence interval
$= 80 + 1.96\frac{20}{\sqrt{100}}$	$= 80 - 1.96\frac{20}{\sqrt{100}}$
$= 80 + 3.92$	$= 80 - 3.92$
$= 83.92$	$= 76.08$

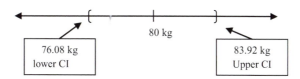

The width of the confidence interval for the mean is affected by the following:

Confidence level
- The higher the confidence level, the wider the interval.

$$95\% \text{ confidence level:constant}(z) = 1.96 \rightarrow X \pm 1.96 \frac{s}{\sqrt{n}}$$

$$99\% \text{ confidence level:constant}(z) = 2.58 \rightarrow X \pm 2.58 \frac{s}{\sqrt{n}}$$

Variance (σ) in the population
- Variance measures how far a set of (random) numbers spreads out from their average value.
- The greater the variance, the wider the interval.

Number of cases (n)
- The larger the number of cases, the narrower the interval.

Other confidence intervals
- Confidence interval for the difference between two proportions.
- Confidence interval for the difference between two means.
- Confidence interval for relative risk.
- Confidence interval for odds ratio.
- Confidence interval for standard deviation.

Further literature

Carroll SR, Carroll DJ. Statistics made simple for school leaders. Illustrated ed. Rowman & Littlefield; 2002. ISBN 9780810843226.

Diagnostic testing

An important part of medical research is to develop and improve diagnostic testing. Diagnostic testing is essential in medicine to gain information regarding a patient's disease status.

A good diagnostic test should have:

- A positive test result in a sick person.

- A negative test result in a healthy person.

Diagnostic tests such as imaging procedures or laboratory tests are usually not error-free and contain uncertainties. Statistical methods are used to quantify the uncertainties. The **sensitivity** and **specificity** is a statistical measure of the performance of a diagnostic test (Table 4.2).

TABLE 4.2 Calculation of sensitivity, specificity.

		Patient	
		Diseased	Disease-free
Test	Positive result	**True positive**	**False positive**
	Negative result	false negative	true negative

		Patient		
		Diseased	Disease-free	
Test	Positive result	a	b	$a + b$
	Negative result	c	d	$c + d$
Total		$a + c$	$b + d$	N

Sensitivity
- Probability of recognizing a diseased person as diseased.
- SENSITIVITY = number of true positive/numbers of diseased.
  $$= \frac{a}{a + c}$$
  SENSITIVITY = number of false negatives/numbers of diseased.
  $$= \frac{c}{a + c}$$

Specificity
- Probability to recognize a disease-free person as disease-free.
- SPECIFICITY = number of correct negatives/numbers of disease-free people
  $$= \frac{d}{b + d}$$
  SPECIFICITY = number of false positives/number of disease-free people
  $$= \frac{b}{b + d}$$

Example
Fecal occult blood test and colon cancer.

		Patient	
		Colon cancer	Healthy
Fecal occult blood test	Positive	73	111
	Negative	233	1680
	Total	306	1791

Sensitivity

$$= \frac{a}{a+c} = \frac{73}{306}$$
$$= 23.9\%$$

= *24 out of 100 patients with colon cancer are detected with the fecal occult blood test as having colon cancer.*

Specificity

$$= \frac{d}{b+d} = \frac{1680}{1791}$$
$$= 93.8\%$$

= *94 out of 100 healthy (disease-free) patients are recognized as colon cancer free with the fecal occult blood test.*

Likelihood ratio

Question: Is the fecal occult blood test a good diagnostic test?

→ The likelihood ratio is used to assess a test.

A measure for assessing a test is the probability quotient (LR +) for a positive test:

LR + = SENSITIVITY/1 − SPECIFICITY
= Proportion of sick people with a positive test/Proportion of healthy people with a positive test.

Interpretation: How many times more likely is a positive test result in sick people in relation to healthy people.

The probability quotient (LR −) for a negative test is:

LR − = 1 − SENSITIVITY/SPECIFICITY
= Proportion of diseased people with a negative test/Proportion of healthy people with a negative test.

Interpretation: How many times less likely is a negative test result in diseased people in relation to healthy people?

With a **sensitivity** of 50% and **specificity** of 50%, the probability of being correct is 50%. So just as high as when guessing or flipping a coin.

- Moderate evidence is five times better than guessing.
- Conclusive evidence is ten times better than guessing.

LR +	LR −	Interpretation
>10	<0.1	Conclusive
5−10	0.1−0.2	Moderate evidence
2−5	0.2−0.5	Small evidence
1−2	0.5−1	Insignificant

Jaeschke et al.[i]

Relationship between sensitivity and specificity (Fig. 4.12)

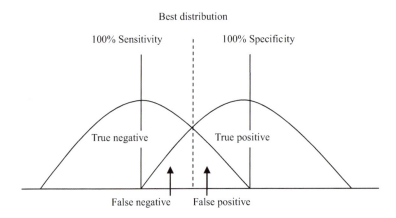

FIGURE 4.12   Sensitivity and Specificity.

Left shift

- Sensitivity ↑ = True positive ↑, false positive ↑
- Specificity ↓ = True negative ↓, false negative ↓

Positive predictive value and negative predictive value
- Sensitivity and specificity is the ability of a test to correctly identify the disease and the disease-free.

Clinically it is more relevant to know:

- Is a patient with a positive test result truly diseased?
- Is a patient with a negative test result truly disease-free?
- This can be calculated using the positive predictive value and negative predictive value.

Example

HIV test.

When the HIV test was first developed, after each positive HIV test a second HIV test was necessary to decide whether someone was truly infected with HIV.

The HIV test has a sensitivity of 99.5% and a specificity of 99.8%. This means that the test recognized 99.5% of those infected with HIV as truly diseased and 99.8% of those who are not infected as truly disease-free.

If all 80 million residents in Country A are tested for HIV, despite the high sensitivity of the test, there would be a probability of 0.2% to have a false positive result. That would be 160,000 people with a false positive result. In comparison, there are around 60,000 people living with HIV in Country A. This means that there are more false positive results than there are infected people. This is due to the low HIV prevalence of around 0.0008.

Positive predictive value = PPV
Probability of a test positive individual to truly being diseased
Bayes rule:

$$PPV = \frac{Sensitivty * Prevalence}{Sensitivity*Prevalence + (1 - prevalence)(1 - Specificity)}$$

Negative predictive value = NPV
Probability of a test negative individual to actually be disease-free
Bayes rule:

$$NPV = \frac{Specificity*(1 - Prevalence)}{Specificity*(1 - Prevalence) + (1 - Sensitivity)*Prevalence}$$

Example

	Cancer	Cancer free (healthy)	
Fecal occult blood test—positive	73	111	**184**
Fecal occult blood test—negative	223	**1680**	**1913**
Total	306	1791	2097

PPV = number of true positives / numbers of test positives
= 73/184 = 39.7%

With a positive test result, only 39.7% of those who test positive have actually cancer!

NPV = number of true negatives/numbers of test negatives
= 1680/1913 = 87%

With a negative test result, 87% of those who test negative are truly healthy.

Prevalence & PPV/NPV
- Positive and negative predictive values depend on the prevalence of a disease.
- Even when the sensitivity and specificity of a test is high, both PPV and NPV are low with a low prevalence of a disease.

Example with a prevalence of 5%

	Cancer	Healthy	
Fecal occult blood test—positive	25	124	149
Fecal occult blood test—negative	80	1868	1948
Total	105	1992	2097

Prevalence = 105/2097 = 5%
Sensitivity = 25/105 = 23.9%
Specificity = 1868/1992 = 93.8%
PPV = 25/149 = 16.8%
NPV = 1868/1948 = 95.9%

Example with a prevalence of 50%

	Cancer	Healthy	
Fecal occult blood test—positive	251	65	316
Fecal occult blood test—negative	798	983	1781
Total	1049	1048	2097

Prevalence = 1049/2097 = 50%
Sensitivity = 25/105 = 23.9%
Specificity = 1868/1992 = 93.8%
PPV = 251/316 = 79.4%
NPV = 983/1781 = 55.2%

The sensitivity and specificity of the test did not change, but the PPV and NPV change depending on the prevalence of the disease.

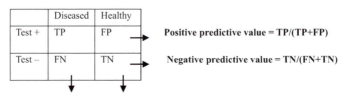

	Diseased	Healthy
Test +	TP	FP
Test −	FN	TN

Positive predictive value = TP/(TP+FP)

Negative predictive value = TN/(FN+TN)

Sensitivity = TP/(TP + FN) Specificity = TN/(TN + FP)
Efficacy and effectiveness
Efficacy

- The effectiveness of treatment in the "ideal world" of controlled studies (under ideal conditions).

Effectiveness

- Effectiveness refers to its performance under "real-world" conditions.

Measure of association

Risk factor	Disease	
	+	−
+	a	b
−	c	d

Relative risk = RR
- Relative risk is a ratio of the probability of an event occurring in the exposed group versus the probability of the event occurring in the nonexposed group.
- The relative risk estimates the strength of association between exposure and outcome.
- It is the measure of association for a cohort study (Case-control study- = odds ratio).
- It describes the absolute change in risk.

$$\text{Relative risk} = \frac{\text{Incidence risk of exposed}}{\text{Incidence risk of nonexposed}} = \frac{a/a+b}{c/c+d}$$

Interpretation

RR = 1   No association between exposure and outcome: incidences are the same in both groups.
RR > 1   Positive association: exposure is a risk factor for the outcome.
RR < 1   Negative association: exposure is a protective factor.

Example

Smoking	Lung cancer	
	+	−
+	80	20
−	10	90

$$\text{Relative risk} = \frac{80/100}{10/100} = 8$$

RR = 8, the risk of a smoker getting lung cancer is 8 times higher than the risk of a nonsmoker getting lung cancer.

Odds ratio = OR

- Odds ratio (OR) is a measure of association between an exposure and an outcome.
- OR is the measure of association for case-control studies.
- With small numbers of cases (rare diseases). The interpretation of OR is similar to RR.
- For a larger number of cases (common diseases), OR is higher than RR.
- OR can also be used if no data on incidence is available or RR cannot be calculated.

Risk factor	Disease	
	+	−
+	a	b
−	c	d

$$\text{Odds ratio} = \frac{\text{Number of cases}}{\text{Population} - \text{number of cases}} = \frac{a/c}{b/d} = \frac{a^*d}{c^*b}$$

Interpretation

OR = 1 No association between exposure and outcome: incidences are the same in both groups.

OR > 1 Positive association: exposure is a risk factor for the outcome.

OR < 1 Negative association: exposure is a protective factor.

Example 1

Rare disease:

Smoking	Bladder cancer	
	+	−
+	10	90
−	5	95

$$\text{Odds ratio} = \frac{10/5}{90/95} = \frac{10^*95}{5^*90} = 2.1$$

OR = 2.1, the odds of a smoker getting bladder cancer is 2.1 times higher than the odds of a nonsmoker getting bladder cancer.

$$RR = \frac{10/100}{5/100} = 2$$

In rare diseases (small number of cases), OR is close to RR.

Example 2

Common disease

Smoking	Lung cancer	
	+	−
+	80	20
−	10	90

$$\text{Odds ratio} = \frac{80/10}{20/90} = \frac{80*90}{10*20} = 36$$

$$RR = = \frac{80/100}{10/100} = 8$$

With frequent illnesses (large number of cases), OR is larger than RR.

Attributable risk = AR

- *Attributable risk describes the proportion of illnesses that are most likely to be attributed to a particular exposure in the population.*
- *It considers the risk of the nonexposed population to be affected by the illness (risk of exposed persons).*
- *It measures the impact of a risk factor.*
- *It measures of the importance for the association between risk factor and outcome.*
- *It indicates by how much you can reduce or prevent the incidence of illness if you would eliminate the risk factor.*
- *It is usually calculated as the difference between the incidence of the exposed and that of the unexposed:*

AR = IE (incidence in exposed group) − IN (incidence in not exposed group)

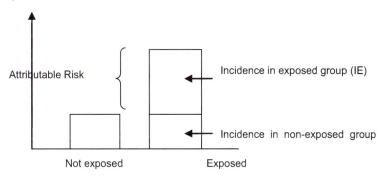

$$\text{Attributional risk} = \frac{a}{a+b} - \frac{c}{c+d}$$

Example

Smoking   Lung cancer

	+	−
+	80	20
−	10	90

$$\text{Attributional risk} = \frac{80}{80 + 20} - \frac{10}{10 + 90} = 0.7$$

Interpretation: The risk of developing lung cancer can be reduced by 70% (from 80% to 10%) by quitting smoking.

Attributable risk percentage = AR%

- *AR% is the percentage of incidence in the disease of the exposed group caused by the exposure.*
- *Specifies the percentage by which the incidence of disease can be reduced or prevented if the risk factor is eliminated.*

Example

Exposed group → lung cancer incidence in smoker: 100/100000
Nonexposed group → lung cancer incidence in nonsmoker: 20/100000

$$AR\% = AR\% = \frac{100 - 20}{100} \cdot 100 = 80\%$$

- *80% of lung cancer incidence is caused by smoking.*
- *80% of lung cancer incidence can be prevented if the risk factor "smoking" is eliminated.*

Population attribute risk = PAR

- Population attributable risk (PAR) is the proportion of the incidence of a disease in the population (exposed and unexposed) that is due to exposure.
- It is the incidence of a disease in the population that would be eliminated if exposure were eliminated.
- Important from the public health perspective.
- PAR helps with policy making in healthcare and public health.

$$\text{Population attributable risk} = \text{Incidence}_{\text{Population}} - \text{Incidence}_{\text{nonexposed}}$$
$$= AR \cdot \text{Prevalence}_{\text{Exposed}}$$

Population attribute risk percent = PAR%

- PAR% is the percentage of the incidence of a disease in the population that could be prevented if the exposure were completely eliminated.

$$PAR\% = \frac{\text{Incidence}_{\text{Population}} - \text{Incidence}_{\text{nonexposed}}}{\text{Incidence}_{\text{Population}}} \cdot 100$$

$$PAR\% = \frac{PAR}{\text{Incidence}_{\text{Population}}} \cdot 100$$

Absolute risk reduction = ARR = risk difference = RD
- Describes the absolute difference in the incidence (risk) between the exposed and nonexposed group.

Absolute risk reduction = risk of exposed group − risk of nonexposed group.

Example

A blood pressure medication lowers the risk of heart attack from 90% to 45%

$$\text{Absolute risk reduction} = 90\% - 45\%$$
$$= 45\%$$

Relative risk reduction = RRR
- Relative risk reduction describes the relative decrease of the risk (by percentage) of an exposed group compared to an unexposed group.
  Relative risk reduction = relative risk − 1
  = (Risk before intervention − risk after intervention/risk before intervention)

Example 1

$$RR = 0.8 \quad 0.8 - 1 = -0.2 = -20\% \rightarrow \text{a risk reduction of 20\%}$$
$$RR = 3.2 \quad 3.2 - 1 = 2.2 = \text{a risk increase of 220\%}$$

Example 2

Drug A lowers the risk of diabetes from 10% to 7%.
$$RRR = (10\% - 7\%)/10\% = 30\%$$

Absolute risk reduction versus relative risk reduction
- Absolute risk reduction should always be viewed in relation to the relative risk reduction and vice versa.
- Results of a study can be interpreted falsely if AR and RR are not presented together.

Example

Same RRR but different ARR
  Study A and B both show a relative risk reduction of 50% for myocardial infarction (RR = 0.5)

The absolute numbers in the studies show the following:

- *Study A: from 80% to 40% → **absolute risk reduction** = 40%*
- *Study B: from 4% to 2% → **absolute risk reduction** = 2%*

Change in ARR with unchanged RRR.

	ARR (%)	RRR (%)
80% → 40%	40	50
50% → 25%	25	50
4% → 2%	2	50

Example

Same ARR but different RRR

Study A and B both show an absolute risk reduction of 10% for myocardial infarction

The relative numbers in the studies show the following:

- *Study A: from 11% to 1% → relative risk reduction = 0.09*
- *Study B: from 55% to 45% → relative risk reduction = 0.82*

Change in RRR with unchanged ARR.

	ARR (%)	RRR (%)
11% → 1%	10	90
50% → 40%	10	20
90% → 80%	10	11

Number need to treat = NNT

- Number need to treat is a measure of how many patients need to be treated in order to expect an effect on one patient.
- A negative NNT is shown as number needed to harm (NNH).
- NNT is an important measure in statistics to estimate the effect and frequency of adverse outcome of a treatment.

$$\text{NNT} = \frac{1}{\text{Absolute risk reduction}} = \frac{1}{\text{ARR}}$$

Example

A blood pressure medication lowers the risk of heart attack from 10% to 6%.

$$
\begin{aligned}
\textit{Absolute risk reduction (ARR)} \quad &= 10\% - 6\% = 0.1 - 0.06 \\
&= 4\% = 0.04
\end{aligned}
$$

$$NNT = \frac{1}{4\%} = \frac{1}{0.04} = 25$$

25 patients need to be treated to prevent a heart attack in one patient.

Number need to harm = NNH

- Number need to harm is a measure of how many people need to be treated (or exposed to a risk factor) in order for one person to have a particular adverse effect.
- It is similar to NNT, but instead of the effect the adverse effect is calculated

Example

A blood pressure drug shows 10% impotence as a side effect in the I intervention group and 6% in the placebo group.

$$NNT = \frac{1}{6\%} = \frac{1}{0.06} = 16.666$$

When 17 patients are treated with the blood pressure medication, one patient becomes impotent.

Endnote

i. Jaeschke R, Guyatt GH, Sackett DL. Users' guides to the medical literature. III. How to use an article about a diagnostic test. B. What are the results and will they help me in caring for my patients? The Evidence-Based Medicine Working Group. JAMA 1994;271(9):703−7.

Chapter 5

Planning a research study

Chapter outline

Planning a research study (Fig. 5.1)

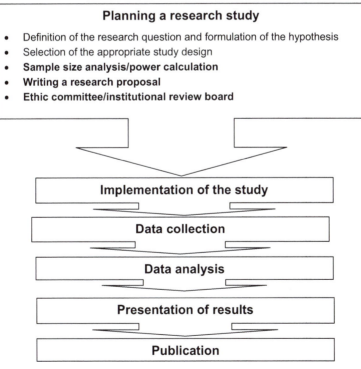

FIGURE 5.1 Planning a research study.

- The planning of a research study starts with an idea of the researcher or scientist.

The Practical Guide to Clinical Research and Publication.
DOI: https://doi.org/10.1016/B978-0-12-824517-0.00016-2
© 2021 Elsevier Inc. All rights reserved.

- A well thought out research plan is important and will serve as a solid foundation of the study.
- A poor study plan can lead to numerous systematic errors resulting in low internal and external validity of the study.
- A poor study design cannot be corrected afterwards.
- It is important to discuss the research planning with different specialists in that field and to revise it multiple times before finalizing it.

Writing a research proposal
- The purpose of writing a research proposal is to demonstrate the intellectual vision and aspirations of the researcher and a well conducted plan.
- A research proposal must address the following questions:
  1. What is the main title?
  2. The main research question. (What do I want to study? What am I trying to accomplish?)
  3. The background to the study. (Why is the topic important?)
  4. A brief background literature review. (Has similar research being conducted before?)
  5. A proposed methodology. (How will I conduct my research?)
  6. A proposed time schedule. (What is the schedule for the project from beginning to end?)

Research question

- To formulate a research question extensive knowledge on that particular topic is required.
- An appropriate research question can only be worked out if there is enough knowledge of the topic and the current research trend.
- A literature and database search to that particular topic is strongly encouraged.
- Expert consultation or mentorship may be required.

A research question should be
1. **Clear**: Specific and detailed enough so that the reader can easily understand the purpose.
2. **Focused**: Narrow enough that it can be answered thoroughly.
3. **Concise**: Brief but comprehensive.
4. **Novel**: A new concept or approach.
5. **Original**: The principal investigator should synthesize an original concept with his unique knowledge that is not available in the same form from previous studies.
6. **Knowledge contribution**: What is already known about that topic? What is the new knowledge gain with this research question?

The research question is the single most important part in a study design!

Each clinical trial must have a primary question. The primary question, as well as secondary or subsidiary questions, should be carefully selected, clearly defined, and stated in advance (Lawrence, 1998).[i]

PICO
Formulating a research question after the PICO criteria[ii]

- The PICO criteria (population, intervention, control, and outcome) developed by McMaster University is a helpful tool for creating a structured research question.
- It should help to present the research question systematically and clearly.
- The cochrane collaboration recommends the use of the PICO criteria in the process of formulating a research question (Table 5.1).
- A good research question is precise and well-defined and can be obtained using pre-existing research methods.

TABLE 5.1 Formulating a good and poor research question.

	Good research question	Poor research question
Population	CAD with >70% stenosisPatients between 60 and 70 years	Heart-sick people
Intervention	1 h treadmill every day at 5 km/h	Sports
Control	No treadmill	No sport
Outcome	Heart attack confirmed by EKG and troponin	Heart attack

Primary outcome
- The primary outcome measure is the outcome that an investigator considers to be the most important among the many outcomes that are to be examined in the study.

Secondary outcome
- The secondary outcome measure is the planned outcome measure in the protocol that is not as important as the primary outcome measure, but is still of interest in evaluating the effect of an intervention.
- Most clinical studies have more than one secondary outcome measure.

Example
Question: Does Metformin 850 mg daily reduce diabetes-related retinopathy?

Primary outcome: diabetes-associated retinopathy

Secondary outcomes
- *Blood pressure*
- *Blood parameters*
- *Other diseases associated with diabetes (e.g., nephropathy, neuropathy)*

Hypothesis

Hypothesis
- A hypothesis is a specific predictive statement, testable assumption, or explanation that then will be tested through a research study or experimentation.
- It is a particular property of a population, such as presumed differences between groups on a particular variable or relationships between variables.

Null hypothesis (H_0)
- A null hypothesis is a type of hypothesis that proposes that there is no difference or relationship between two measured phenomena or no association between groups of a particular variable.

Alternative hypothesis (H_1)
- The alternative hypothesis is the hypothesis used in hypothesis testing that is contrary to the null hypothesis.
- It is usually consistent with the research **hypothesis** because it is constructed from the literature review, previous studies, previous knowledge, etc.

Interpretation of hypothesis
- A null hypothesis (H_0) is never "accepted." It is either "rejected" or "failure to reject."
- The distinction between "acceptance" and "failure to reject" is best understood in terms of confidence intervals.
- Failing to reject a hypothesis means a confidence interval contains a value of "no difference."

It is incorrect to accept or prove a hypothesis. A hypothesis can only be rejected or fail to reject.

Example

Null hypothesis: Drug A does not lower blood pressure.
   Alternative hypothesis: Drug A lowers blood pressure.

- Neither the null hypothesis nor the alternative hypothesis is actually 100% correct.

   One-sided hypothesis
   H_0:A > B, H_1:A ≤ B

- If there is a strong belief that the study intervention has a one-sided effect, a one-sided hypothesis can be formulated.
- If the research direction is one-sided, the hypothesis can be formulated one-sided.
- If a one-sided hypothesis is formulated, a small number of sample size is necessary (Fig. 5.2).

Example

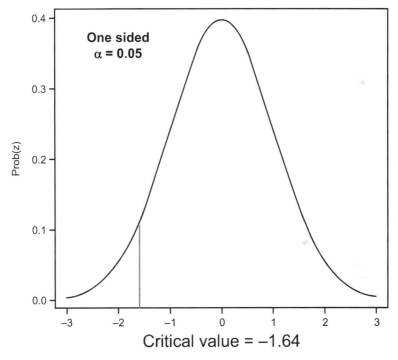

FIGURE 5.2   One-sided hypothesis.

Null-hypothesis: Drug A lowers the blood pressure.
   Two-sided hypothesis
   H_0: A = B, H_1: A≠B

- A two-sided hypothesis is advantageous because it is generally difficult to predict in which direction the relationship (positive or negative) between two measured phenomena is.
- The results and conclusion of a two-sided hypothesis provides more information than a one-sided hypothesis.

- If a two-sided hypothesis is formulated, a higher sample size is needed (Fig. 5.3).

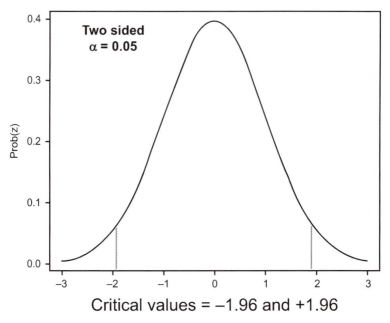

FIGURE 5.3   Two-sided hypothesis.

Example

Null-hypothesis: Drug A has an influence on (lowers or raises) blood pressure.

α **and** β **errors of the null-hypothesis**

		Reality	
		H_0 is true	H_0 is not true
Decision	Fail to reject H_0	Correct decision	β **error** (Type II error)
	Reject H_0	α **error** (Type I error)	**Correct decision (Power)**

α **error (type 1 error)**
- A statistically significant difference is found, although in reality it does not exist (wrongly rejecting the null-hypothesis).

- The probability to reject the null hypothesis, although the null-hypothesis is true.
- To falsely describe an ineffective therapy as effective (consumer risk).

β errors (type 2 errors)
- No statistically significant difference is found, although in reality a difference exists (wrongly fail to reject the null hypothesis).
- The probability of not rejecting the null-hypothesis, even though the null-hypothesis is false.
- Not recognizing an effective therapy as effective (producer risk).

Power $(1 - \beta)$
- "Power" is the probability of rejecting the null hypothesis if it is false.
- To recognize an effective therapy as effective.
- **A high "power" is what the researcher ideally wants to achieve in a research study**.

Example

H: Drug A has no influence on blood pressure.
   H: Drug A lowers blood pressure.

		Reality	
		H_0 is true	H_0 is not true
Decision	Fail to reject H_0	H_0 is "accepted" and in reality, drug A has no influence on blood pressure. **correct decision**	H_0 is "accepted" although in reality drug A lowers blood pressure. **β error**
	Reject H_0	H_1 is "accepted" although in reality drug A has no effect on blood pressure. **α error**	H_1 is "accepted" and in reality, drug A lowers blood pressure. **correct decision**

Study protocol

All research studies should be carefully planned before they are carried out. The study protocol is a document that describes all aspects of a study in detail. All relevant information about the study must be specified before the start of the study. There are international guidelines, but mostly institutions have their own templates for the study protocol. After completion of the study protocol, it will be submitted to the responsible institutional review board (IRB), ethics committee, or approval authority (Table 5.2).

TABLE 5.2 Sample of a study protocol.

Study protocol	
Title page	• Contains the study title and the name and address of the institutes involved.
Summary	• Overview of the main aspects of the study.
Ethical aspects	• Notes on the ethics committee, patient information, and declaration of consent.
Administrative	• Name, profession, and function of all persons involved in the implementation of the study.
Introduction	• Scientific background and justification for carrying out the study.
Goal of the study	• Study scientific question (formulated as hypothesis).
Study design	• Description of the study design (e.g., observational study, randomization), targeted number of patients, and the centers involved.
Time schedule	• Key dates of the study (start, interim analysis, and completion).
Study population	• Description of the participants in the study (criteria for inclusion and exclusion, e.g., age, sex, and comorbidity).
Implementation	• Detailed schedule of the study (possibly with graphics).
Methods	• Description of the data to be recorded as well as the examination methods and measuring instruments.
Dropout	• Give reasons for the early termination of the study. • Possibility of leaving the study at the request of the participant.
Therapy safety	• Procedure with undesirable events (side effects).
Data management	• Description of the structure of a database and data entry.
Data protection	• Description of the specific measures on data protection and confidentiality.
Quality assurance of the data	• Monitoring, audit, and other measures to ensure the correctness of the data collected.
Case number estimation, statistical analysis	• Calculation of the required number of participants and determination of the statistical analysis methods.
Reporting	• Establishing protocols, interim reports, and final report. • Planned publications in scientific journals.

(Continued)

TABLE 5.2 (Continued)

Study protocol	
Bibliography	• List of all scientific literature used in the manuscript.
Attachment	• Sample of questionnaires, patient information, patient consent, and physician information.

Source: Courtesy of Charite University Medicine, Berlin. http://www.kks.charite.de/Deutsch/
Informationen/Patienten/Aufklaerungsposter/Studienprotokoll.pdf.

Study registration

- A study register is a platform for registering research studies before they are carried out (Table 5.3).

TABLE 5.3 Registry for studies.

National institutes of health (USA)	http://www.clinicaltrials.gov
EU clinical trials register	http://www.clinicaltrialsregister.eu
International clinical trials registry platform (ICTRP) (WHO)	http://www.who.int/ictrp/en
DRKS (German register for clinical studies)	http://www.germanctr.de https://drks-neu.uniklinik-freiburg.de/drks_web
Biomed central (UK)	ISRCTN.org
Britain's national research register	http://www.doh.gov.uk
BMC	http://www.biomedcentral.com
Australian New Zealand clinical trials registry (ANZCTR)	http://www.anzctr.org.au
Chinese clinical trial register	http://www.chictr.org
Clinical trials registry—India	http://www.ctri.nic.in

- Most IRBs and journals require all clinical trials to be registered before patient enrollment.
- The definition of a "clinical trial" is not uniform but usually includes any study that has prospective patient enrollment.

Aim of a study registration
- Ensure transparency in clinical research.
- Make studies accessible to the public.
- Avoidance of a change in the primary or secondary study hypothesis and outcome measures.
- Avoidance of falsifying studies.
- Most major journals will not accept a manuscript submission if the study was not registered before the study began (Table 5.3).

Sample size

Estimating a sample size

- A sample size estimation is essential to obtain a valid study result.
- The sample size estimation is based on the statistical analysis of the outcome of the study (precision, prevalence, proportion, mean, etc.)
- When planning a study it should be defined how and with which methods the results will be analyzed statistically.
- The methods of sample sizes calculation and the methods of the statistical analysis must match.
- Sample size calculation is also important for economic and patient safety reasons.
- It is important to minimize the number of patients needed that are exposed to an intervention of a study.
- Consider loss to follow up in the sample size calculation. For example, if 5% of the patients will be dropped-out during the study, this 5% should be added in the sample size calculation before patient enrollment.
- A sample size is mandatory in writing a study protocol and for the IRB submission.
- Several sample size calculation software are available (Table 5.4).

TABLE 5.4 Sample size calculation software.

Programs	Costs	Origin
PASS (Power analysis & sample size)	Charge	United States
nQuery advisor	Charge	United States
Epi info	Download/freeware	Centers for Disease Control and Prevention (CDC), USA
http://www.rad.jhmi.edu/jeng/javarad/samplesize/	Online/freeware	John Hopkins Hospital, USA
http://www.openepi.com	Online/freeware	Emory University, Rollins School of Public Health, USA
http://www.stat.uiowa.edu/~rlenth/Power/index.html	Online/freeware	University of Iowa, USA
http://statpages.org/	Online/freeware	Private website

Example

Inadequate sample size:

   If two out of four people in a population are diseased, the prevalence is 50%. However, due to the small number of cases, no reliable statement can be made reflecting the general population.

Necessary factors for sample size calculation

- Primary outcome.
- Distribution of the outcome.
- Number of groups.
- Hypothesis.
- Statistical test used.
- Expected effect/precision (difference, relative risk, odds ratio, prevalence, etc.).

Factors influencing sample size

- α and β errors
- Variability
- Effect size

		Reality	
		H0 is true	H0 is not TRUE
Decision	H0 not reject	Correct decision	**β error** (Type II error)
	Reject H0	**α error** (Type I error)	**Correct decision (Power)**

Influence of α and β on sample sizes

- Small α error: more patients required.
- Small β error (= high power): more patients required.

Variability: how do the values spread

- Small variability → fewer patients required.
- Large variability → many patients required.

Effect of the outcome

- Small outcome effect → many patients required
- Great outcome effect → fewer patients required

In medicine, a confidence interval of 95% ($\alpha = 0.05$) and a power of 80% are commonly used.
   CI 95% → $\alpha = 0.05$ → $z_{1-\alpha/2} = 1.96$
   Power 80% → $\beta = 20\%$ → $z_{1-\beta} = 0.84$

Sample size calculation for a proportion
- A sample size calculation for a proportion is based on the confidence interval for the proportion.
- The equation for the confidence interval is converted into an equation for the sample size calculation.
- If the estimated proportion of the intervention is unclear, 50% can be used (provides the maximum number of cases).

Confidence interval for a proportion =
- p = frequency/proportion
- $z_{1-\alpha/2}$ = quantile of the standard normal distribution (e.g., for a 95% CI: $z_{1-\alpha/2}$ = 1.96)
- $z_{1-\alpha/2}$ = 1.96 (value of the 95% confidence interval → α = 0.05)
- n = sample size

Conversion by number of cases (n):

$$n = \frac{(z_{1-\alpha/2})^2}{\delta^2} \cdot p(1-p)$$

Example

Study B attempts to evaluate the incidence of the side effects of drug A.
Estimated value: 5% side effect p = 0.05
Precision: ± 2% δ = 0.0 2
Significance level α: 5% $z_{1-\alpha/2}$ = 1.96

$$n = \frac{(1.96)^2}{0.02^2} \cdot 0.05(1-0.05) = \frac{3.8416}{0.0004} \cdot 0.05 \cdot 0.95 = 456.19$$

457 patients are required

Number of cases when comparing two proportions
- The sample size calculation for two proportions is based on the statistical test for two proportions.

Conversion by number of cases (n):

$$n_{\text{pro Gruppe}} = \frac{(z_{1-\alpha/2}\sqrt{2\bar{p}(1-\bar{p})} + z_{1-\beta}\sqrt{p_1(1-p_1) + p_2(1-p_2)})^2}{(p_1-p_2)^2}$$

$$\bar{p} = \frac{p_1 + p_2}{2}$$

- p_1: proportion of group 1
- p_2: proportion of group 2
- $\bar{p}$: proportion of both groups
- $z_{1-\alpha/2}$, $z_{1-\beta}$: Quantile of the standard normal distribution

1. $z_{1-\alpha/2} = 1.96$ (value of the 95% Confidence interval $\rightarrow \alpha = 0.05$)
2. $z_{1-\beta} = 0.84$ (Power 80% $\rightarrow \beta = 20\%$)
3. $= 1.28$ (Power 90% $\rightarrow \beta = 10\%$)

Simplified equation (Lehr, 1992)[iii]
- $\alpha = 0.05$, power 80%

$$n = 16 \cdot \frac{\overline{\pi}(1 - \overline{\pi})}{(p_1 - p_2)^2}$$

Example

Study A is evaluating the relationship of lung cancer and smoking.

Heart attack in smoker (group 1): 20% $p_1 = 0.2$
Heart attack in non-smokers (group 2): 10% $p_2 = 0.1$
Heart attack in both groups: 15% $\overline{p} = 0.15$
Significance level α: 5% $z_{1-\alpha/2} = 1.96$
Power: 80% ($\beta = 20\%$) $z_{1-\beta} = 0.84$

$$n_{\text{pro Gruppe}} = \frac{(1.96\sqrt{2\cdot0.15(1-0.15)} + 0.84\sqrt{0.2(1-0.2)+0.1(1-0.1)})^2}{(0.2-0.1)^2}$$

$= 200.4$
$= 201$ in each group or 402 in total
Simplified formula

$$= 16 \cdot \frac{0.15 \cdot 0.85}{0.01} = 204$$

$= 201$ in each group or 402 in total

Sample size calculation for a mean
- Is derived from the confidence interval for the mean value

$$\text{Confidence interval} = X \pm z_{1-\alpha/2} \frac{\sigma}{\sqrt{n}}$$

- $\sigma =$ estimated standard deviation
- $z_{1-\alpha/2} =$ quantile of the standard normal distribution
- $z_{1-\alpha/2} = 1.96$ (value of the 95% confidence interval $\rightarrow \alpha = 0.05$)
- $n =$ sample size
- The confidence interval equation is converted into an equation for the number of cases (n):

Conversion to a number of cases, number of cases (n):

$$n = \frac{z_{1-\alpha/2}^2 \cdot \sigma^2}{\delta^2}$$

Example

- *Measurement of blood sugar levels in a group of diabetes patients.*
- *Estimated $\sigma = 200$ mg/dL $\sigma = 200$*
- *Precision: ± 50 mg/dL $\delta = 50$*
- *Significance level α: 5% $z_{1-\alpha/2} = 1.96$*
- $n = \frac{1.96^2 \cdot 200^2}{50^2} = \frac{3.84 \cdot 40000}{2500} = 61.44 \approx 62 \, people$

Sample size when comparing two means

- The sample size calculation for comparing two means is based on confidence interval (CI) for the difference between two means.

Conversion by number of cases (n):

$$n_{\text{per group}} = \frac{(z_{1-\alpha/2} + z_{1-\beta})^2 \cdot 2\sigma^2}{\delta^2}$$

- $\sigma =$ estimated standard deviation
- δ: estimated difference of the mean values
- $z_{1-\alpha/2}$, $z_{1-\beta}$: quantiles of the standard normal distribution
  1. $z_{1-\alpha/2} = 1.96$ (value of 95% confidence interval $\rightarrow \alpha = 0.05$)
  2. $z_{1-\beta} = 0.84$ (Power 80% $\rightarrow \beta = 20\%$)
  3. $= 1.28$ (Power 90% $\rightarrow \beta = 10\%$)

Simplified formula (Lehr, 1992)

$\alpha = 0.05$, power 80%

$$n_{\text{pro group}} = \frac{(z_{1-\alpha/2} + z_{1-\beta})^2 \cdot 2\sigma^2}{\delta^2}$$

$$= \frac{(1.96 + 0.84)^2 \cdot 2\sigma^2}{\delta^2}$$

$$= \frac{(2.8)^2 \cdot 2\sigma^2}{\delta^2}$$

$$= \frac{(7.84) \cdot 2\sigma^2}{\delta^2}$$

$$= \frac{2 \cdot (7.84) \cdot \sigma^2}{\delta^2}$$

$7.84 \approx 8$

$$n = 16 \cdot \frac{\sigma^2}{\delta^2}$$

Example

A study A is trying to investigate the difference in body weight in group 1 and group 2.

Estimated body weight in group 1 (mean) 120 kg
Estimated body weight in group 2 (mean) 100 kg
Estimated difference of the mean 20 kg
Standard deviation 40 kg
Significance level α: 5% $z_{1-\alpha/2} = 1.96$
Power: 80% $z1 - \beta = 0.84$

$$n_{\text{per Group}} = \frac{(z_{1-\alpha/2} + z_{1-\beta})^2 \cdot 2\sigma^2}{\delta^2}$$

$$= \frac{(1.96 + 0.84)^2 \cdot 2 \cdot 40^2}{20^2}$$

$$= \frac{7.84 \cdot 2 \cdot 1600}{400}$$

62.72 patients in each group or 125 in total
Simplified formula

$$n = 16 \cdot \frac{\sigma^2}{\delta^2}$$

$$= 16 \cdot \frac{40^2}{20^2}$$

= 64 in each group or 128 total.

Endnotes

i. Lawrence F. Fundamentals of clinical trials. New York: Springer; 2015.
ii. Aslam S, Emmanuel P. Formulating a researchable question: a critical step for facilitating good clinical research. Indian J Sex Transm Dis AIDS 2010;31:47−50.
iii. Lehr R. Sixteen S-squared over D-squared: a relation for crude sample size estimates. Stat Med 1992;11(8):1099−102.

Chapter 6

Study design

Chapter outline

Classification of clinical studies (Fig. 6.1)

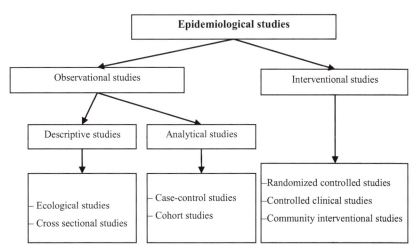

FIGURE 6.1 Classification of clinical studies.

The Practical Guide to Clinical Research and Publication.
DOI: https://doi.org/10.1016/B978-0-12-824517-0.00014-9

Observational studies

- Observational studies are where the researcher observes the effect of a risk factor, diagnostic test, treatment, or other interventions without trying to make any intervention to the participating population. Cohort studies and case control studies are two types of observational studies. Although observational studies are more prone to confounding and bias, they can be a very useful tool in epidemiology as there may be important practical or ethical issues that preclude the design of an randomized controlled trials (RCT) in certain questions. In general, use of an adequate large sample size and appropriately sampled data in observational studies allows for statistical adjustment for most measured confounding factors.

Descriptive studies

- Descriptive studies are observational studies that describe the characteristics of the population or phenomenon that is being studied.
- In other words, descriptive studies primarily focus on describing the nature of a demographic segment, without focusing on "why" a certain phenomenon occurs.
- Descriptive studies describe the patterns of disease occurrence in relation to variables such as person, place and time. (e.g., prevalence, mortality rate, birth rate, fertility rate, disease frequency etc.)

Analytical studies

- Analytical studies attempt to identify the relationships between diseases and their causes/exposure by testing specific hypotheses.
- Samples of subjects are identified and information about exposure status and outcome is collected.
- In analytical studies groups of subjects are compared in order to estimate the magnitude of association between exposures and outcomes.

Descriptive studies

Ecological studies

- An ecological study is an observational study that is characterized by trying to relate exposure and disease at the region and population level, rather than at the individual level.
- Ecological studies are often used to measure prevalence and incidence of disease, particularly when disease is rare.

Cross-sectional studies (Fig. 6.2)

- Cross-sectional studies are types of observational studies in an empirical study (e.g., survey, content analysis) that is carried out, or data is collected at one given point in time.
- A cross-sectional study is entirely descriptive.
- A descriptive cross-sectional study assesses how frequently, widely, or severely the variable of interest occurs throughout a specific demographic.

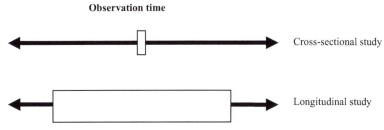

FIGURE 6.2   Cross-sectional study and longitudinal study.

Analytical studies

Observational studies

Cohort study & case control study

- In observational studies, the exposure and outcome are observed over a certain period of time and the association is described (Fig. 6.3 and 6.4).

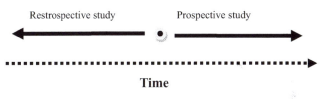

FIGURE 6.3   Prospective and retrospective studies.

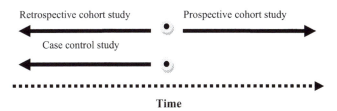

FIGURE 6.4   Prospective and retrospective cohort studies.

- No interventions are carried out by the examiner.
- Although observational studies are more prone to confounders and bias, compared to interventional studies, they are a very useful tool in epidemiology since practical or ethical matters can preclude the design of an RCT with certain research questions.

Advantage
- Less expensive and easier to carry out than intervention studies.
- Exposure and outcome can be linked in relation to time.
- Ethically less limitations compared to interventional studies.

Disadvantage
- The investigational exposure can be influenced by unknown factors.
- Observational studies are prone to recall bias.
- Observational studies are prone to Neyman bias.
- In observational studies, confounders are unevenly distributed.
- A long observational period is required for diseases that appear late after exposure. e.g., cancer.

Prospective studies
- Data is collected prospectively after the study is planned. (e.g., questionnaire)
- Prospective cohort study or randomized controlled studies are prospective studies.

Advantage
- Data can be collected specifically focused and targeted to the research question.
- Data quality can be improved with good study planning.

Disadvantage
- Ethically challenging research data cannot be collected.
- It is time consuming as data collection requires a certain collection and follow-up time.

Retrospective studies
- Data is collected and stored during before the study was planned without a specific research question (e.g., electronic medical record).

Advantage
- In retrospective studies, research questions can be answered for which a prospective study does not exist or cannot be carried out for ethical reasons.
- It is relatively inexpensive compared to a prospective study, since the data pool is already available.

Disadvantage
- In retrospective studies, certain factors (bias) cannot be controlled, or only with difficulty.
- Since the data collection took place before the study planning, the quality of the available data is not always good.
- Data quality cannot be improved since the dataset already exists.
- Additional data cannot be collected.

Cohort study (Fig. 6.5)

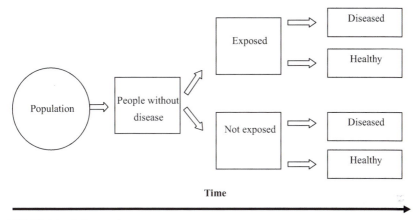

Time

FIGURE 6.5   Cohort study.

- A cohort study can be performed prospectively or retrospectively.
- It examines the association between a given exposure (risk factor) and the outcome (disease).

Advantage
- Ethically safe.
- A cohort study is generally easier to perform and less expensive than intervention study.

Disadvantage
- Large numbers of cases or long follow-up times are necessary for rare diseases.
- There must be an exposure for the disease.
- The exposure may be influenced by a hidden variable (confounder).
- A randomization is not possible.
- No "blinding" available.
- Observational studies are prone to selection bias and reporting bias.

Example
Smoking causes lung cancer. 1000 people are examined, including 500 smokers (Fig. 6.6).

Case control study

Case control study
- The case control study is a retrospective observational study (Fig. 6.7).

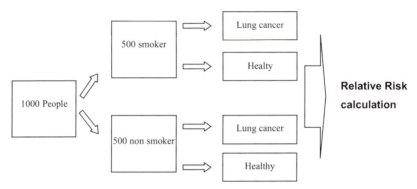

FIGURE 6.6   Example of a cohort study.

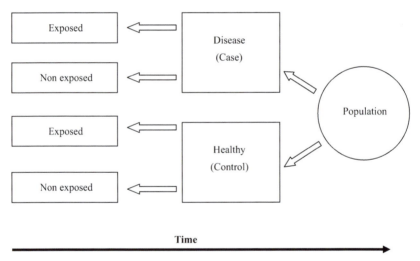

FIGURE 6.7   Case control study.

- A target event (e.g., lung cancer) is defined as a case and a suitable control group (e.g., no lung cancer) is created.
- The target and control groups are evaluated retrospectively about the presence of an exposure (smokers, nonsmokers, asbestos exposure...).
- The effect ratio "odds ratio" is calculated.

Advantage
- Well-suited study design for rare diseases.
- It is easier and less expensive than interventional studies.
- Less cases are needed compared to a cohort study.

Disadvantage
- Finding an appropriate control group is not always easy.

- Susceptible to selection bias and reporting bias.
- Control group matching requires more complicated statistical analysis.
- Matching is usually only possible for a few variables (age, gender, and important additional risk factors).
- There is a risk of overmatching. (Matching for factor that is not a confounder).
- There is a risk of data loss. A case cannot be used if no appropriate control is identified.
- The influence of the matching variables cannot be evaluated.

Example

Behcet disease: Behcet disease is a rare disease, causing vascular inflammation in numerous organs, including ulceration of the mouth, genital mucosa and involvement of the eyes. The cause is still unknown with an incidence of 0.6 cases per 100,000 people.

With a prevalence of 0.6−100,000, one would have to examine a cohort (population) of 10,000,000 people in 60 cases. This would hardly be feasible. In a case control study, the 60 cases are collected and a control group that is similar in all relevant parameters of the case group is created. These are then compared (Fig. 6.8).

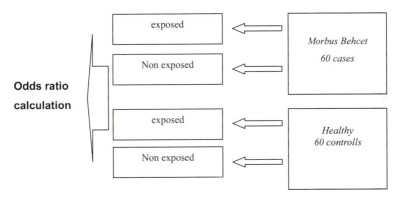

FIGURE 6.8   Figure of a case control study.

Selection of cases and controls
- Cases and controls should be as similar as possible in all relevant parameters.
- The only difference variable should be the outcome of the study.

Matching
- Matching is the selection of one or more controls for each case based on defined parameters.
- Age and gender are often used for matching.
- The goal of matching is to reduce the confounding factors.
- The statistical significance of the study can be increased.

Matching strategies

Individual matching

- For each case, a control is selected based on specific matching variables.
- Controls are selected so that they are similar to the cases in all important characteristics.
- Matching can be done as 1:1, or with multiple controls per case (1:*n*).

Example

For a 50-year-old male case, a 50-year-old male control is matched.

Frequency matching

- Frequency matching is a sampling design used in case−control studies to assure that cases and controls have the same distributions over strata defined by matching factors.
- The number of controls is selected according to the number of cases within a matching variable

Example

For each category of the matching variables, the number is prepared following the number selected to controls at cases

Age (years)	Cases (N)	Controls (N)
0−20	70	70
21−40	80	80
41−60	60	60

Mantel-Haenszel method

- The Mantel-Haenszel method is an important method in case-control studies to control confounders
- It provides a "combined" odds ratio for the "matched" groups

$$OR_{MH} = \frac{\sum_{i=1}^{K} a_i \cdot d_i / n_i}{\sum_{i=1}^{K} b_i \cdot c_i / n_i}$$

$K =$ Number of strata

Residual confounding

- It is possible that there is a different distribution of the variables in each group (Fig. 6.9).

Nested case-control studies

- A nested case control study is a case control study within an existing cohort (cohort study)

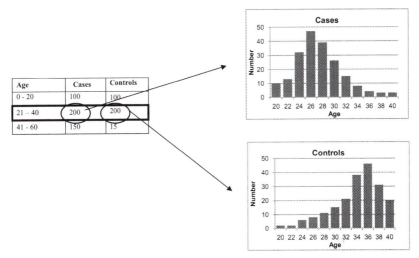

Age	Cases	Controls
0 - 20	100	100
21 – 40	200	200
41 - 60	150	15

FIGURE 6.9   Residual confounding.

- Cases within the cohort are compared to healthy controls from the cohort.
- The characteristics of the participants in the case and control group are similar because both were selected for the overall "cohort"
- This reduces the risk of a selection bias.

Case-cohort study
- Cases: all cases within an existing cohort.
- Control: random sample of the whole cohort as a control group (including cases).

Intervention studies

Intervention studies
- Interventional studies are often prospective and are specifically designed to evaluate direct impacts of treatment or preventive measures on disease.
- In contrast to observational studies, the exposure is determined or assigned by the examiner.
- The "**Intervention**" it defined and established by the study investigator (for example, medication, treatments, and surgeries).

Advantage
- Since the exposure is determined by the examiner, there is no need to search for an exposed group, which is difficult or impossible with rare exposures. (e.g., new medication, new surgical technique, and new treatment method).

Disadvantage
- Not every research question can be carried out as an intervention study.

- It is ethically incorrect to test dangerous substances as human exposure and to withhold the effectiveness of proven medication.
- Intervention studies are expensive and require more resources than observational studies.

Randomized controlled trials

Randomized controlled trials

RCT are the gold standard in medicine

- RCT are studies in which people are allocated at randomly to receive a clinical intervention or a control intervention. (intervention or control group)
- Randomization reduces bias and provides a rigorous tool to examine cause-effect relationships between an intervention and outcome.
- In clinical research, RCTs are the best way to study the safety and efficacy of new treatments.

Advantage
- Best clinical study design to evaluate efficacy and causality.
- Even distribution of confounders (confounding factors) through randomization.
- Biased can be further minimized with allocation concealment and blinding.
- Smaller sample size is needed compared to observational studies.

Disadvantage
- Costly and complex to implement a RCT.
- Sometimes difficult to enroll participants that meet the study criteria.
- Certain research questions cannot be performed with RCTs due to ethical reasons. e.g., an effective therapy should not be withheld from patients.

RCT types
Simply randomized controlled trial (Fig. 6.10)

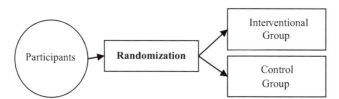

FIGURE 6.10   Simply randomized controlled trial.

Randomized controlled crossover study
- Each participant receives all interventions during the study (Fig. 6.11).

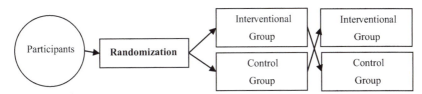

FIGURE 6.11 Randomized controlled crossover study.

Advantage
- All participants receive the same intervention.
- Fewer subjects are required.
- Minimize systematic errors.

Randomized controlled factorial study
- Two studies imbedded in one study (Fig. 6.12).

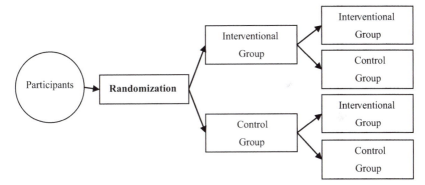

FIGURE 6.12 Randomized controlled factorial study.

Randomization
- The randomization is based on the statistical theory of random samples.
- The group assignment of subjects is done randomly.
- Randomization methods: computer generated, throw dice.

Objective and advantage of randomization
- Each study participant has the same probability of being assigned to the intervention or the control group.
- All known and unknown confounders become evenly distributed!
- This largely ensures that the two groups differ only in terms of the intervention.

Randomization methods
- Individual randomization: individuals are assigned to the respective group randomly.
- Block randomization: subjects are divided into blocks before the start of the study.
- For example 3 subjects in one block. The randomization is carried out between the individual blocks.
- Cluster randomization: randomizations are performed in specific groups. (e.g., schools, hospitals, cities. . .)

No randomization

In studies without randomization several other factors may affect the study results.

- Different patient selection between the groups.
- Different data acquisition between the groups.
- Time dependent effects.
- Placebo effect.
- Other effects.

Without randomization the effect is overestimated by 16%–33%, which is not caused by random variability.

Blinding (=blinding, masking)
- Open: no blinding.
- **Simply blinded**: the study participants are blinded. The subject does not know which treatment he is receiving.
- **Double blinded**: participants and investigators are blinded. In addition to the participant, even the study investigator does not know which intervention he is performing on the patient.
- **Triple blinded**: participants, examiner and evaluator/interpretation are blinded.

Aim of blinding
- Reduces distortion/bias during intervention and the measurement of the outcomes.

Performance bias
Systematic difference in the treatment of the groups (beside from the intervention).

Example
The treating doctor unconsciously treats the patient differently. (e.g., conducts more extensive physical examinations with the intervention group).

Allocation concealment
- "Allocation concealment" means the assignment of participants to each study group is concealed.
- The examiner should not know in which group the participant will be assigned to, until the intervention takes place.
- If the assignment is not concealed, there is a risk of conscious or unconscious influence of the examiner, which could lead to manipulation of the assignment of the next subject.

---

no blinding: effect is overestimated by 17%−19%
no allocation concealment: effect is overestimated by 33%−41%

Intention to treat analysis (ITT)
- All subjects who took part in the study are evaluated at the end
- That includes participants that drop out during the study (on patient request, other causes)
- ITT analysis reflects closer the reality. Because similar to ITT, in reality a proportion of patients do not follow a therapy properly or discontinue it early.

Per protocol analysis (PP)
- Only the subjects who completed the study will be evaluated.
- Drop out subjects are excluded from the evaluation.
- PP analysis represents the optimal condition, but does not reflect the reality.

Conducting a randomized controlled trial

The following steps should be observed and documented when carrying out the study.

- Inclusion and exclusion criteria for patients.
- Main outcome measure.
- Intervention.
- Statistic evaluation methods.
- Collected variables (e.g., standard laboratory values such as blood tests, urine tests, liver function tests and specific measurements of biomarkers etc.).
- Exclusion criteria for a patient.

The following flowchart is helpful for orientation (Fig. 6.13).

Literature analytical studies

Literature-analytical-studies

- Since a single epidemiological study can never definitively answer the research question, all available evidence must be taken into account. Literature analytical studies are secondary studies that summarize and evaluate primary studies (Fig. 6.14).

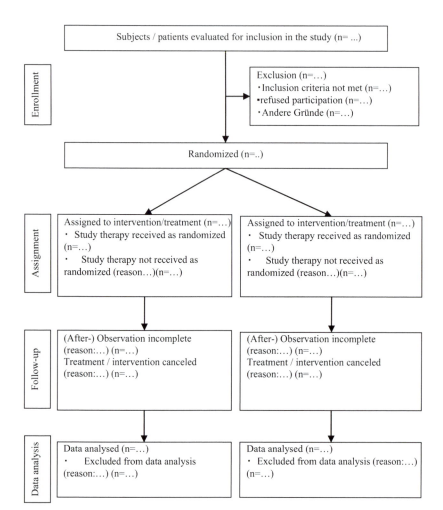

FIGURE 6.13   Randomized controlled trial flowchart.

Systematic reviews

- A systematic review is a scientific research review article in which all available primary studies are systematically identified to a clearly formulated research question (Table 6.1).
- Their quality of each included study is assessed and the results are summarized (secondary research).
- A systematic review has the highest level of evidence and is basis for evidence-based medicine implemented medical care.
- Some, but not all, systematic reviews lead to a *meta*-analysis.

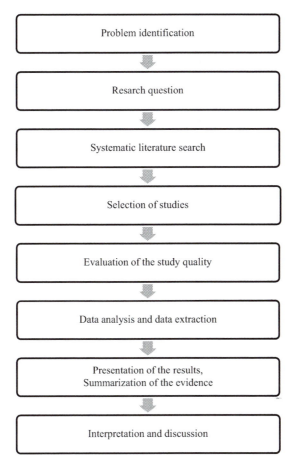

FIGURE 6.14   Flow diagram of the methodology for creating a systematic review.

TABLE 6.1 Cochrane standard for a systematic review.[ii]

- Background
- Objectives
- Criteria for considering studies for this review
  - Types of studies
  - Types of participants
  - Types of interventions
  - Types of outcome measures
- Search strategy for identification of studies
- Description of studies-methodological quality of included studies
- Results
  - Characteristics of included studies
  - Characteristics of excluded studies
  - Comparisons and data
- Discussion of results

Aim of a systematic review
- To increase the statistical significance of the results.
- The resolution of ambiguities between studies with the same research question.
- To evaluate contradicting results from different studies.
- To evaluate a research questions that was not considered of an individual randomized controlled trial (e.g., subgroups).

Limitation
- Not all studies are published: It is difficult to include unpublished studies in a systematic review.
- Not all studies are registered: Some studies cannot be found through internet search.
- If the methodological quality of a single study is poor, it also affects the quality of a systematic review.
- Publication bias impacts a systematic review (studies with positive results are published more often).
- Language bias has impacts on a systematic review.

Problem identification
- If there is no summarizing literature available to a research question (systematic reviews, *meta*-analysis), the necessity of a systematic review can be considered.

Question
- A research question is formulated based on the PICO scheme (population, intervention, comparison, outcome).
- Individual terms are precisely defined.
- Inclusion and exclusion criteria as well as primary and secondary outcome measure are defined

Example (Table 6.2)

TABLE 6.2 Definition of inclusion criteria for a systematic review.

Criteria	Inclusion	Exclusion
Study design	• Only randomized controlled intervention studies (RCT)	• No explicitly named or recognizable study design • Observational studies, reviews, prevalence/incidence studies, guidelines • Clearly nonspecialist articles • No abstract available

(Continued)

TABLE 6.2 (Continued)

Criteria	Inclusion	Exclusion
Population	• Patients with impaired glucose tolerance (IGT) who were analyzed by test procedures before the start of the study. • Age: no limit • Gender (male and female)	• Patients with diagnosed diabetes • Embryo, fetus • No impaired glucose tolerance • IFG diagnosis only. • Studies with animals
Intervention	• Intervention "lifestyle intervention" • Affected at least one of the IDF lifestyle factors	• Interventions not designated as "lifestyle intervention" • None of the interventions influencing the IDF lifestyle factors • pure drug studies • Secondary and tertiary prevention
Controls	• Control group with minimal intervention (intervention group accordingly) • Ideal: no intervention	• Lack of a control group or comparison option • Noncomparable control groups (e.g., diet vs drug lowering blood pressure)
Outcome	Primary: incidence of diabetesSecondary: • Mortality, morbidity, QALY, • Clinical parameters (weight, blood pressure, blood sugar. . .) • Follow-up observation> 6 months	• Lack of quantifiable patient-oriented endpoints • Follow-up <6 months

Systematic literature research

How to perform an electronic database research (PubMed)
• Develop an appropriate search strategy for the research question.
• Define the databases or sources to be searched (Table 6.3).

TABLE 6.3 List of bio-medical databases.

Database	Website
PubMed (MEDLINE)	http://www.pubmed.com
EMBASE	http://www.embase.com
Cochrane	http://www.cochrane.org
NLM (National Library of Medicine)	http://www.nlm.nih.gov/
NCBI (National Center for Biotechnology Information)	http://www.ncbi.nlm.nih.gov/

- Define the study design and the study duration.
- Develop a search strategy.
  1. Define the search terms.
  2. Search for synonyms (possibly truncation/wildcards use n (*))
  3. Test search terms individually (in PubMed the "Query Translation" can be checked under "Details" (shows the exact scope and extent of a search word))
  4. Keywords identification (MeSH terms)
  5. Logical combination of search words (AND/OR)
  6. "Limit" setting
  7. Test search strategy
- Carrying out a "pre-search"
- Improvement/optimization of the search strategy

Secondary literature
- Use the "Related articles" function in PubMed.
- Search the reference list of included studies for other relevant studies.

Query translation

Example 1

*Free text search term: **body mass index***
Query Translation: "body mass index" [MeSH Terms] OR ("body" [All Fields] AND "mass" [All Fields] AND "index" [All Fields]) OR "body mass index" [All Fields]
*   The "Query Translation" function, shows that the search terms also automatically contain MeSH terms.*

Example 2

*Free text search term: **Lifestyle intervention***
Query Translation: ("life style" [MeSH Terms] OR ("life" [All Fields] AND "style" [All Fields]) OR "life style" [All Fields] OR "lifestyle" [All Fields]) AND intervention [All Fields]
*   The "Query Translation" function, shows that the search terms automatically include other search terms.*

Truncation/wildcards (*)
- Truncation is a search method in which symbols are used in place of letters or words to help you broaden your search.
- If an asterisk (*) is added to the end of a phrase, truncation is performed.

Example

*Free text search term: prediabet**
Query Translation: prediabet [All Fields] OR prediabeta [All Fields] OR prediabete [All Fields] OR prediabetec [All Fields] OR prediabeteic [All Fields]

OR prediabetes [All Fields] OR prediabetes/diabetes [All Fields] OR prediabetes/ifg [All Fields] OR prediabetes/metabolic [All Fields] OR prediabetes/ newly [All Fields] OR prediabetes/t2dm [All Fields] OR prediabetes' [All Fields] OR prediabeteszhez [All Fields] OR prediabeti [All Fields] OR prediabetic [All Fields] OR prediabetic/diabetic [All Fields] OR prediabetic/prehypertensive [All Fields] OR prediabetic '[All Fields] OR prediabetica [All Fields] OR prediabeticas [All Fields] OR prediabetice [All Fields] OR prediabetiche [All Fields] OR prediabeticheskie [All Fields] OR prediabeticheskikh [All Fields] OR prediabeticheskimi [All Fields] OR prediabetici [All Fields] OR prediabetickem [All Fields] OR prediabeticky [All Fields] OR prediabetickych [All Fields] OR prediabetico [All Fields] OR prediabetics [All Fields] OR prediabetics' [All Fields] OR prediabetics [A ll Fields] OR prediabetin [All Fields] OR prediabetique [All Fields] OR prediabetiques [All Fields] OR prediabetiske [All Fields] OR prediabetnoto [All Fields] OR prediabetom [All Fields] OR prediabetu [All Fields] OR prediabetychnymy [All Fields]

Selection of studies (Fig. 6.15)
- At least two independent expert or evaluator.
- Literature selection according to the defined inclusion and exclusion criteria.
    1. Title Analysis: Everything should be blinded except the title (author, institution, journal, database, abstract).
    2. Abstract analysis: Everything except the title and abstract should be blinded (author, institution, journal, database)
    3. Full-text analysis: Author, institution, journal and database should be blinded.
- If there is a disagreement among the reviewers, discuss extensively each detail for the inclusion/exclusion criteria and/or add a third expert.
- Use flowchart to be able to trace each step easily.
- Present the results of the reviewers in a four-field table and evaluate the discrepancies (interrater reliability) according to Kappa.

Example

Cohen's Kappa
- The kappa value evaluates the number of matches between two raters.
- The equation for Cohen's Kappa is:

		Reviewer 2		
		+	−	
Reviewer 1	+	P_{++}	P_{+-}	P_{+}
	−	P_{-+}	P_{--}	P_{-}
		P_{+}	P_{-}	

$$K = \frac{Po - Pe}{1 - Pe}$$

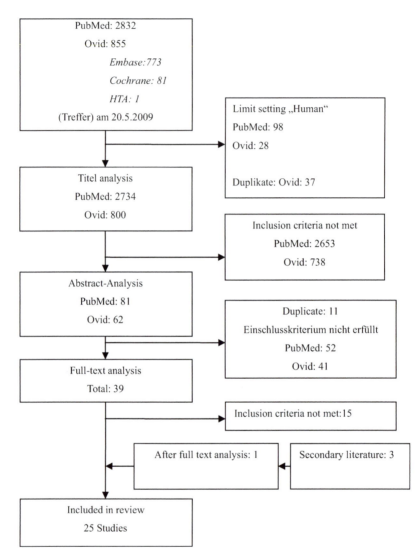

FIGURE 6.15   Flowchart for study selection.

Po = value of the observed matches

$$= P_{++} + P_{--}$$

Pe = value of the random matches

$$= P_+P_+ + P_-P_-$$

- If the raters agree in all of their judgments, $K = 1$.
- If the raters disagree in all of their judgments $K = 0$.

There are different classifications for interpreting the kappa values (Table 6.4).

TABLE 6.4 Interpretation of the Kappa value according to Landies and Koch.[i]

K	Interpretation	
<0	No agreement	No agreement
0.0−0.20	Slight agreement	Some agreement
0.21−0.40	Fair agreement	Adequate agreement
0.41−0.60	Moderate agreement	Mediocre agreement
0.61−0.80	Substantial agreement	Significant agreement
0.81−1.00	Almost perfect agreement	Almost perfect match

Example (Tables 6.5 and 6.6)

$$Po = P_{++} + P_{--} = \frac{23}{39} + \frac{12}{39} = 0.897 \approx 0.90$$

$$Pe = P_{+}P_{+} + P_{-}P_{-} = \frac{26}{39} \cdot \frac{24}{39} = 0.67 \cdot 0.62 + 0.33 \cdot 0.38 = 0.54$$

$$K = \frac{Po - Pe}{1 - Pe} = \frac{0.90 - 0.54}{1 - 0.54} = 0.78$$

TABLE 6.5 Four-field table for the kappa calculation after full-text analysis.

		Reviewer 2		
		+	−	
Reviewer 1	+	23	1	24th
	−	3rd	12th	15
		26	13	39

TABLE 6.6 Kappa value according to COHEN (full text analysis).

	Value	95% confidence interval (lower-upper)
Po	0.90	0.76−0.97
Pe	0.54	−
K	0.78	0.57−0.98

Evaluation of the study quality
- The methodology and study quality of the included studies are analyzed using predefined quality assessment instruments, criteria or checklists (Table 6.7).

TABLE 6.7 Instrument for study quality evaluation.

Instrument	Application
Sign 50	Methodology Checklist 1: Systematic reviews and *Meta*-analysis Methodology Checklist 2: Randomized controlled trials Methodology Checklist 3: Cohort studies Methodology Checklist 4: Case-control Studies Methodology Checklist 5: Diagnostic studies
NHS CASP (critical appraisal skills program)	12 questions to help you make sense of a diagnostic test study 11 questions to help you make sense of a case control study 12 questions to help you make sense of a cohort study 10 questions to help you make sense of RCT 10 questions to help you make sense of reviews
Jadad scale (Oxford scale)	RCT
IQWIG	Quality assessment: diagnostic studies

Data analysis and data extraction
- The included studies are used to analyze the predefined outcomes.
- Data is analyzed and compiled.

Presentation of the results, summarizing the evidence
- The extracted data are presented in tables and Figure.
    1. Specify the searching period.
    2. Overview of the included studies (author, title, year, journal, country, language, and impact factor)
    3. Population of the studies included (age, gender, BMI, and ethnicity)
    4. Intervention of the included studies (Which intervention was carried out in the respective study?)
    5. Control of the included studies (How was the control group in each study?)
    6. Outcomes of the included studies (What outcomes were found in the studies?)

Interpretation and discussion
- Interpretation and discussion of the results.
- Discussion of possible bias and discussion of generalizability.
- Discussion of future research approach.

Meta-analysis

A *Meta*-analysis is a quantitative, formal, epidemiological study design with the statistical procedure for combining data from multiple studies. It is used to systematically assess previous research data to derive a conclusion for a specific research question. Decisions about the validity of a hypothesis cannot be based on the results of a single study because results typically vary from study to study. *Meta*-analyses can be a challenging, requiring large resources and statistical understanding. The outcomes from a *meta*-analysis includes a more precise estimate of the hypothesis than any individual study contributing to the pooled analysis (Fig. 6.16).

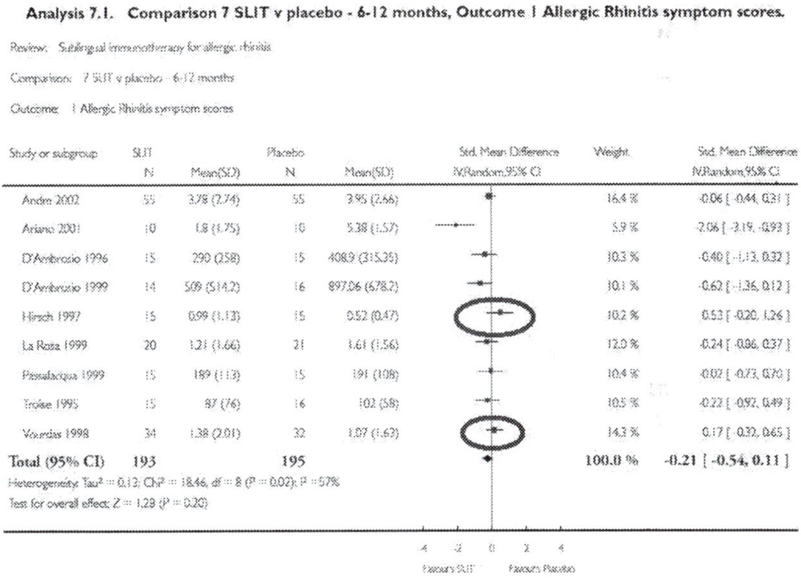

Analysis 7.1.   Comparison 7 SLIT v placebo - 6-12 months, Outcome 1 Allergic Rhinitis symptom scores.

Review: Sublingual immunotherapy for allergic rhinitis

Comparison: 7 SLIT v placebo - 6-12 months

Outcome: 1 Allergic Rhinitis symptom scores

Study or subgroup	SLIT N	Mean(SD)	Placebo N	Mean(SD)	Std. Mean Difference IV,Random,95% CI	Weight	Std. Mean Difference IV,Random,95% CI
Andre 2002	55	3.78 (2.74)	55	3.95 (2.66)		16.4 %	-0.06 [-0.44, 0.31]
Ariano 2001	10	1.8 (1.75)	10	5.38 (1.57)		5.9 %	-2.06 [-3.19, -0.93]
D'Ambrosio 1996	15	290 (258)	15	408.9 (315.36)		10.3 %	-0.40 [-1.13, 0.32]
D'Ambrosio 1999	14	509 (514.2)	16	897.06 (678.2)		10.1 %	-0.62 [-1.36, 0.12]
Hirsch 1997	15	0.99 (1.13)	15	0.52 (0.47)		10.2 %	0.53 [-0.20, 1.26]
La Rosa 1999	20	1.21 (1.66)	21	1.61 (1.56)		12.0 %	-0.24 [-0.86, 0.37]
Passalacqua 1999	15	189 (113)	15	191 (108)		10.4 %	-0.02 [-0.73, 0.70]
Troise 1995	15	87 (76)	16	102 (58)		10.5 %	-0.22 [-0.92, 0.49]
Vourdas 1998	34	1.38 (2.01)	32	1.07 (1.62)		14.3 %	0.17 [-0.32, 0.65]
Total (95% CI)	**193**		**195**			**100.0 %**	**-0.21 [-0.54, 0.11]**

Heterogeneity: Tau² = 0.13; Chi² = 18.46, df = 8 (P = 0.02); I² =57%

Test for overall effect: Z = 1.28 (P = 0.20)

-4   -2   0   2   4

Favours SLIT   Favours Placebo

FIGURE 6.16   Example of a *meta*-analysis: effectiveness of sublingual immunotherapy in allergic rhinitis (Wilson Dr)[v]

- Individual studies, including RCTs, can deliver different results on the same research.
- A summary of the available data including a scientific analysis is therefore necessary.
- The fundament of a *meta*-analysis is a systematic review.
- Like a systematic review, the *meta*-analysis summarizes all relevant studies to one research question.
- The data and result is then summarized and analyzed statistically in order to have a conclusive statement the specific research question.

- PRISMA (Preferred reporting items for systematic reviews and *meta*-analyses) aims to help authors improve the reporting of systematic reviews and *meta*-analyses.[iii]
- MOOSE (**M**etaanalysis **o**f **o**bservational **s**tudies in **e**pidemiology) is a checklist that contains specifications for reporting of *meta*-analyses of observational studies in epidemiology and is useful for authors, editors, and reviewer.[iv]

Benefits of a meta-analysis
- The results are much more accurate and reliable than a single study result.
- Effect variations between the studies can be identified.
- A *meta*-analysis can identify publication bias.

Problem
- Heterogeneity: Some of the identified and included studies differ so much in their clinical characteristics that a comparison is difficult.
- Poorly conducted single studies can lead to inaccurate results of a *meta*-analysis.

Example

- If one were to cite the circled studies individually, they would incorrectly interpret a positive effect.

Identifying of randomized controlled trials
- Randomized controlled studies are often used for systematic review or *meta*-analysis.
- The following search strategies show how to selectively identify RCT in PubMed.

1. Simple strategy for the researcher with little time

```
1. Randomized controlled trial [pt] *
2. Animals [mh] *
3. Humans [mh]
4. # 2 NOT (# 2 AND # 3) *
5. # 1 NOT # 4
```

2. Simple strategy with increased sensitivity and acceptable precision

```
1. Clinical trial [pt]
2. Animals [mh]
3. Humans [mh]
4. # 2 NOT (# 2 AND # 3)
5. # 1 NOT # 4
```

3. Strategy with high sensitivity (CRD/cochrane, revision 2005)

---

1. Clinical trial [pt]
2. Randomized [from] *
3. Placebo [from]
4. Clinical trials [mh]
5. Randomly [ab]
6. Trial [ti] *
7. # 1 OR # 2 OR # 4 OR # 5 OR # 6
8. Animals [mh]
9. Humans [mh]
10. # 8 NOT (# 8 AND # 9) *
11. # 7 NOT # 10

[pt] denotes publication type

[ab] denotes a word in the abstract

[mh] denotes medical subject headings (MeSH)

[ti] denotes a word in the title

Sets 2−4 (in strategies 1 and 2) and sets 8−10 (strategy 3) capture animal studies that are not also human studies and allow these records to be safely excluded from the search, while returning records that are not indexed as either human or animal studies, as these may be relevant.

4. Search strategy with the maximum sensitivity: Highly Sensitive Search Strategy (HSSS) RECOMMENDATION!

---

1. RANDOMIZED CONTROLLED TRIAL.pt.
2. CONTROLLED CLINICAL TRIAL.pt.
3. R ANDOMIZED CONTROLLED TRIALS.sh.
4. R ANDOM ALLOCATION.sh.
5. D OUBLE-BLIND METHOD.sh.
6. S INGLE-BLIND METHOD.sh.
7. or/1−6
8. ANIMAL.sh. not HUMAN.sh.
9. 7 Not 8
10. CLINICAL TRIAL.pt.
11. EXP CLINICAL TRIALS
12. (clin adj25 trial $). ti, ab.
13. ((single or double or treble or triple) adj25 (blind $ or mas $)). ti, ab.
14. PLACEBOS.sh.
15. placebo $.ti, from.
16. random $.ti, from.
17. RESEARCH DESIGN.sh.
18. or/10−17
19. 18 not 8
20. 19 not 9
21. COMPARATIVE STUDY.sh.

---

22. exp EVALUATION STUDIES /
23. FOLLOW UP STUDIES.sh.
24. PROSPECTIVE STUDIES.sh.
25. (control $ or prospectiv $ or volunteer $). ti, ab.
26. or/21−25
27. 26 not 8
28. 2 7 not (9 or 20)
29. 9 or 20 or 28

In these examples, upper case denotes controlled vocabulary and lower case denotes free text terms. Search statements 8, 9, 19, and 27 could be omitted if your search takes too long a time to run

5. **Search strategy with the maximum sensitivity to find systematic reviews**

1. REVIEW, ACADEMIC.pt.
2. REVIEW, TUTORIAL.pt.
3. *META*-ANALYSIS.pt.
4. *META*-ANALYSIS.sh.
5. systematic $ adj25 review $
6. systematic $ adj25 overview $
7. *meta*-analy $ or metaanaly $ or (meta analy $)
8. or/1−7
9. ANIMAL.sh. not HUMAN.sh.
10. not 9

Search statements 9 and 10 could be omitted if your search seems to be taking a long time to run.

Clinical practice guidelines

Clinical practice guidelines are systematically developed statements to assist practitioner and patient decisions about appropriate health care for specific clinical circumstances.

- Guidelines translate best evidence into best practice.
- A well-crafted guideline promotes quality by reducing healthcare variations, improving diagnostic accuracy, promoting effective therapy, and discouraging ineffective—or potentially harmful—interventions.
- Guidelines are developed based on the system of the Association of the Scientific Medical.
- Clinical practice guidelines are developed by multidisciplinary committees using an evidence-based approach, combining the best research available with expert consensus on best practice.
- Depending on the stage of development, guidelines are classified into S1, S2 or S3 (Fig. 6.17).

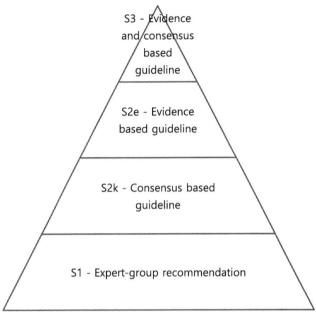

FIGURE 6.17   Clinical practice guideline classification.

- The highest quality level of guidelines is reached in the third stage (S3). These guidelines are developed by a full formalized, systematic development process.

Disadvantage
- Guidelines are based on evidence-based medicine and therefore includes publication bias or language bias
- Inclusion of poorly designed primary studies results in poor or wrong guidelines development.
- 70%−90% of the guidelines are S1 (few S2 and S3)
- S3 guidelines are missing for rare clinical diseases, because there are very few primary studies on the subject.

S1
- A representative group of experts from the Scientific Medical Association comes up with a guideline in an informal consensus, which is approved by the executive board of the medical specialty.

S2
- Existing level 1 guidelines are adopted and processed into a level 2 guideline following a formal consensus procedure.
- Formal consensus procedures are nominal group processes, such as Delphi method and consensus conference.

- A discussion of the "evidence" is performed, and the participation of methodologists is helpful in this procedure.
  - S2e—Is based on evidence that includes a systematic review, analysis and inclusion of selected literature.
  - S2k—Is based on a medical specialty board or panel consensus, without a systematic literature review.

S3
- Guidelines that meet all five criteria of the systematic process below.
  1. **Logical analysis (clinical algorithm):** A special logic (clinical algorithm, decision tree): "if-then" logic on a problem-solving path. Guidelines are a prerequisite for disease management.
  2. **Formal consensus process:** A formal and transparent consensus finding with already approved and evaluated processes (e.g., nominal group process).
  3. **Evidence based medicine:** A formal and transparent scientific evidence handling. The systematic monitoring, evaluation and use of current research results as a basis for clinical decision making. Health care is based on evidence, derived from the best available studies.
  4. **Decision** analysis: A formal outcome analysis (overall clinical result) with a clear statement on the clinical relevance (order of significance), using methods of quantitative and qualitative analysis.
  5. **Outcome analysis:** A formal analysis of cost effectiveness: comparison of costs with the same medical outcome.

HTA reports

Health technology assessment

Health technology assessment (HTA) is a multidisciplinary process that summarizes information about the medical, social, economic and ethical issues related to the use of a health technology in a systematic, transparent, unbiased, robust manner. Its aim is to inform the formulation of safe, effective, health policies that are patient focused and seek to achieve best value. Despite its policy goals, HTA must always be firmly rooted in research and the scientific method.[vi]

- A HTA report is based on evidence-based medicine.
- Methodologically it is similar to a *meta*-analysis.
- Mostly randomized controlled studies are included in the analysis of a HTA.
- The literature search for a HTA is much more extensive than a *meta*-analysis.

- To include all available evidence, gray literature, foreign language literature and unpublished literature are extensively searched and analyzed.
- Another big difference compared to a *meta*-analysis is that it includes cost analysis and ethical aspects.
- Criteria such as effectiveness, security and costs are evaluated, taking into account social, legal and ethical aspects.
- The result of an HTA study is usually published as an HTA report (approx. 200−1000 pages)
- An HTA report should primarily serve as a decision-making aid for health policy matters.

Aim
- Healthcare resources are limited and are becoming increasingly scarce and expensive.
- With the increasing numbers of innovative medical developments, there is a strong need to analyze effectiveness and cost-effectiveness.

Advantage
- Possibly the best, most detailed, and available methodology in evidence-based medicine.

Disadvantage
- Extremely complex and slow.
- Publication bias, language bias.
- Poor primary studies have a negative impact on the HTA report.
- Economic research in medicine is still in the development phase

Health economic studies

Cost analysis studies

Health economic evaluation studies
Cost-of-illness-study (COI)
Cost minimization study (CM)
Cost-effectiveness-analysis (CEA)
Cost utility analysis (CUA)
Cost-benefit analysis (CBA)

Cost analysis

Cost analyzes only record the costs associated with the medical measure or technology (i.e. the input) and do not take into account the effects that are achieved by this measure/technology (for example on the patient's state of health). No comparison to a reference object is carried out.

Medical expenses analysis

Cost-of-illness analysis, only records and examines the costs of a specific illness, often from the perspective of society or health insurers. The direct and indirect costs including the follow-up costs are taken into account and are evaluated. The aim of these analysis is to make decision-makers aware of the anticipated costs of a disease and to make estimates for the success of newly developed medicines and medical services. It is also used to find evidence for the meaningful use of research funds in order to make prioritization and allocation.

Cost-cost analysis

Cost-cost analyzes, cost-minimization analysis, are separate cost analyzes of two or more alternative medical measures or technologies and are limited to the analysis, evaluation and comparison of costs in the form resource consumption of the medical measures/technologies in the same context. The benefit (e.g., health-related quality of life) is not considered, since it is assumed that it will be identical for the medical measures/technologies that are compared. The aim is to determine the best cost alternative based on the application factors.

Cost-benefit analysis

In the cost-benefit analyzes, not only the resource consumption (costs) but also the benefits of medical measures or technologies are assessed monetarily and accordingly expressed in monetary units. The monetary benefit assessment is based either on the willingness to pay/acceptance of the users or on the contribution of the effects to increasing human capital. The measure of these analyzes, is the net benefit in monetary units as the difference between benefit and cost.

Cost-effectiveness analysis

In the context of cost-effectiveness analyzes, the costs are recorded and evaluated as resource consumption for the medical measures or technologies that are compared. The benefit gained is described by a single parameter that is measured in its "natural" medical and therefore nonmonetary units (for example, years of life gained). Accordingly, measures can be formed that describe and compare the cost-effectiveness relationships (e.g., comparisons of costs per year of life gained) and represent whether treatment with the measures/technologies to be compared have an influence on the selected benefit parameters. The aim of this analysis is to determine the amount of resource consumption that is required to achieve a certain effect.

Cost-benefit analysis

In cost-benefit analysis, the costs are recorded and evaluated in the same way as in the cost-effectiveness analysis. However, the benefit is assessed in the form of "utility values", with particular attention being paid to the quality of medical services. The concept of "quality-adjusted years of life" (QALYs) has prevailed in health economics. Then an one-dimensional index for the quality of life is determined from the effects of a medical service on different dimensions of health from a patient's perspective. The benefits for medical measures or technologies are formed by offsetting the gains in years of life and quality of life, that is the life is weighted with the assessment of the health-related quality of life of the patient. The results are then cost-benefit ratios, which show the relation of the costs per QALY gained and can be compared with other medical services from different indication areas if necessary, using the outcome measure QALY.

Cost minimization studies

Cost minimization studies also only examine costs, while comparing alternative interventions for a health problem. In order to be able to interpret the results of this type of evaluation in a meaningful way, the effects of the interventions examined must be the same.

Cost-effectiveness analysis

The additional costs and effects (e.g., remaining years of life) of an intervention are compared to a basic alternative; the ratio of these costs and effects is called the cost-effectiveness ratio. This type of evaluation only makes sense if a primary effect category can be determined and defined as such. Other secondary effects will develop differently and could lead to different cost-effectiveness results. Furthermore, only results from studies with the same effect parameter can be compared with each other.

Pharmacological studies

Pharmacological studies are of great importance in determining a drug's effect and safety in humans. After the discovery and development of the drug animal testing is performed in the preclinical phase. The clinical phase of the study is divided into four phases. Phase 1, phase 2, phase 3, and phase 4. A clinical phase of pharmaceutical product is a long-term process and can take several years (Fig. 6.18).

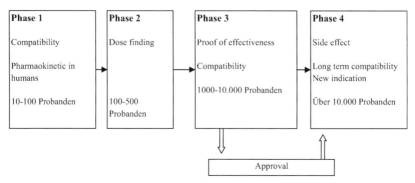

FIGURE 6.18   Pharmacological studies.

Preclinical phase
- Preclinical research to determine the efficacy and safety of the drug.
- Preclinical trials test the new drug on nonhuman subjects for efficacy, toxicity, and pharmacokinetic
- Following pharmacokinetics are tested: Absorption, Distribution, Disposition, Metabolism, & Excretion
- The drug is tested on living organisms or cells, including animals.

Clinical phase
- **Phase I**—In phase I the drug is tested on humans the first time. Less than 100 healthy volunteers will participate to help researchers assess the safety and pharmacokinetics, absorption, metabolic, and elimination effects on the human body, as well as any side effects for safe dosage ranges.
- **Phase II**—Phase II assesses drug safety and efficacy in an 100–500 patients. The optimal dose is analyzed and adverse events and risks are recorded.
- **Phase III**—Phase III includes 1,000–5,000 patients. Phase III trials require extensive collaboration, organization, and follow the Independent Ethics Committee or Institutional Review Board coordination and regulation. Because of their size and comparatively long duration, Phase III trials are the most expensive, time-consuming and difficult trials to design and run.
- **Phase IV**—Phase IV is also known as postmarketing surveillance trial. Following drug approval and manufacturing, the United States Food and Drug Administration (FDA) requires drug companies to monitor the safety of its drug. FDA uses its postmarketing safety surveillance program FDA Adverse Event Reporting System (FAERS). Through this program, manufacturers, health professionals, and consumers report problems with approved drugs.

Endnotes

i. Landis JR, Koch GG. The measurement of observer agreement for categorical data. Biometrics 1977;33:159–74.

ii. https://training.cochrane.org/handbook/current

iii. Moher D, Liberati A, Tetzlaff J, Altman DG; PRISMA Group. Preferred reporting items for systematic reviews and *meta*-analyses: the PRISMA statement. PLoS Med 2009; 21(6): e1000097.

iv. Stroup DF, Berlin JA, Morton SC, Olkin I, Williamson GD, Rennie D, Moher D, Becker BJ, Sipe TA, Thacker SB. *Meta*-analysis of observational studies in epidemiology: a proposal for reporting. *Meta*-analysis Of Observational Studies in Epidemiology (MOOSE) group. JAMA 2000 Apr 19;283:2008−12.

v. Wilson DR, Lima MT, Durham SR. Sublingual immunotherapy for allergic rhinitis: systematic review and *meta*-analysis. Allergy 2005;60(1):4−12.

vi. European Network for Health Technology Assessment. Assessment FAQ. What is health technology assessment (HTA). https://www.eunethta.eu/services/submission-guidelines/ [accessed 01.02.2021].

Chapter 7

Hierarchy of evidence

Chapter outline

Hierarchy of evidence

- A hierarchy of evidence is assigned to studies based on the methodological quality of their design, validity, and applicability to patient care. These decisions give the "grade (or strength) of recommendation" (Fig. 7.1).

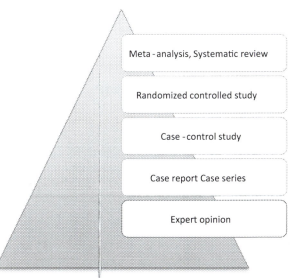

FIGURE 7.1 Hierarchy of evidence.

The Practical Guide to Clinical Research and Publication.
DOI: https://doi.org/10.1016/B978-0-12-824517-0.00010-1

Systematic reviews and meta-analyzes that are based exclusively on randomly controlled studies have the highest significance (level of evidence).

Clinical decisions should be based on meta-analyzes or systematic reviews, never on individual studies.

Recommendation scale according SIGN[i] (Table 7.1)

TABLE 7.1 Evidence hierarchy scale according to Scottish Intercollegiate Guidelines Network (SIGN).[ii]

1++	Meta-analysis, systematic review of randomized controlled trials (RCTs) or randomized controlled trials (RCT)—of high methodological quality, with a low risk of bias.
1+	Well-performed meta-analysis, systematic review or RCT—with a low risk of bias.
1−	Meta-analysis, systematic review or RCT—with considerable risk of bias.
2++	High quality systematic review of case-control studies or cohort studies High-quality case-control studies or cohort studies with a very low risk of confounding or bias and a high probability of causality.
2+	Well-done case-control studies or cohort studies with a small risk of confounding or bias and a medium probability of causality.
2−	Case-control studies or cohort studies with a high risk of confounding or bias and a significant risk that the relationship found is not causal.
3rd	Nonanalytical studies, for example, case reports or case series.
4th	Expert opinion.

1. Levels of evidence 1++ and 1+ studies
2. Levels of evidence 2++ to 1 studies
3. Levels of evidence 2+ to 2++ studies
4. Levels of evidence 2+ to 3.4 studies

Disadvantages

- Although RCTs are the often considered to be the highest level of evidence, not all RCTs are conducted properly and the results should be carefully interpreted.
- RCTs have a high internal validity but a poor external validity.
- Observational studies are being superseded by RCTs as evidence and are considered secondary.
- However, well designed and conducted cohort or case-control studies are not inferior to RCTs.

Recommendation scale according Cox (Table 7.2)

TABLE 7.2 Evidence hierarchy scale according to cox.

Level Ia	Meta-analysis of multiple randomized controlled studies.
Level Ib	Single randomized controlled trial.
Level IIa	Well-planned, nonrandomized controlled trial.
Level IIb	Well-planned experimental study.
Level III	Well-planned nonexperimental study, comparative study, correlation or case-control study.
Level IV	Not evidence-based expert opinion.

Randomized controlled trials versus observational studies. Which one is better?

- **GRADE working group:** "Once the results of high quality randomized trials are available, a few people would argue for continuing to base recommendations on nonrandomized studies with discrepant results" (Atkins et al., 2004).[iii]
- **EBM:** "If the study wasn't randomized, we'd suggest that you stop reading it and go on to the next article in your search" (Sackett et al., 2000, p. 108)[iv].
- **Cochrane collaboration:** In personal correspondence, Julian Higgins of the Cochrane Collaboration replied to the question of whether evidence from RCTs is sufficient, with the following statement "I'm sure there are very many people who subscribe to this view [that RCT evidence is sufficient] (if interpreted as further evidence on the same questions that the RCTs address). Indeed, one might infer this from the fact that the majority of Cochrane reviews include only RCTs. This strongly implies that the authors believe there is no need to look at other evidence (or believe that "Cochrane" thinks they shouldn't look at other types of evidence). I have much sympathy with this, given the numerous unpredictable and largely poorly understood biases in observational studies."
- To answer the question of whether a single well-done RCT trumps evidence from any number of observational studies, Julian Higgins states that "If the RCT was done well, then I would always claim this is either

the right answer or the answer to a different question from the observational studies."

- **SIGN:** The following quote from the SIGN 50 document seems to imply that if there are RCTs, the other evidence need not be considered: "It is also intended to allow more weight to be given to recommendations supported by good quality observational studies where RCTs are not available for practical or ethical reasons."

- **RCTs do not offer better evidence than well-done observational studies** (Worrall, 2002). However, even Worrall admits that RCTs control for at least one potential confounder that current observational studies do not, namely selection bias. But eliminating selection bias may always be important. Observational studies do not necessarily suffer from selection bias; also, the effect of selection bias may be minimal and insufficient to confound the results of the study.[v]

- Even if RCTs provide the best **internal validity**, their **external validity** is often suspect. RCTs are experiments. The experimental setting is often different from general practice. We can't know whether the results of the experiment apply in the real world. RCTs are experiments with volunteers. There are often relevant differences between the population of volunteers and the population that will be treated (Worrall, 2002).

- Because observational studies are not experiments with volunteers, their external validity is often greater than the external validity of RCTs. These issues are important when we consider that sometimes RCTs and observational studies reach different conclusions.

Endnotes

i. https://www.sign.ac.uk/assets/sign_grading_system_1999_2012.pdf

ii. Harbour R, Miller J. A new system for grading recommendations in evidence based guidelines. BMJ 2001;323(7308):334−6.

iii. Atkins D, Best D, Briss PA, Eccles M, Falck-Ytter Y, Flottorp S, Guyatt GH, Harbour RT, Haugh MC, Henry D, Hill S, Jaeschke R, Leng G, Liberati A, Magrini N, Mason J, Middleton P, Mrukowicz J, O'Connell D, Oxman AD, Phillips B, Schünemann HJ, Edejer T, Varonen H, Vist GE, Williams JW Jr, Zaza S; GRADE Working Group. Grading quality of evidence and strength of recommendations. BMJ 2004;19(328):1490.

iv. Sackett DL. Evidence-based medicine: how to practice and teach EBM. Churchill Livingstone, 2000.

v. Worrall J. What evidence in evidence-based medicine? Philos Sci 2002;69(S3):S316−30. [accessed 31.01.2021]. doi:10.1086/341855.

Chapter 8

Funding

Chapter outline

Funding sources

Funding is available from different organizations
- Federal funding
- Private companies
- Nonprofit foundations
- Professional organizations

Federal funding
- http://www.grant.gov
- Grants.gov is one of the largest sources for research funding in the United States.
- It lists all current discretionary funding opportunities from 26 agencies of the United States government, including the National institutes of health (NIH).

National institutes of health
- The NIH Office of Extramural Research is the largest funder of biomedical research in the world.
- NIH funds research in just about every area that's remotely related to human health and disease.
- NIH has 27 Institutes and Centers. Twenty four of them are funding and three of them are non-funding authorities.
- https://grants.nih.gov/grants/oer.htm includes extensive information about NIH grants, and a search function for NIH funding programs.
  1. National Cancer Institute (NCI)—Est. 1937
  2. National Eye Institute (NEI)—Est. 1968
  3. National Heart, Lung, and Blood Institute (NHLBI)—Est. 1948

The Practical Guide to Clinical Research and Publication.
DOI: https://doi.org/10.1016/B978-0-12-824517-0.00013-7

4. National Human Genome Research Institute (NHGRI)—Est. 1989
5. National Institute on Aging (NIA)—Est. 1974
6. National Institute on Alcohol Abuse and Alcoholism (NIAAA)—Est. 1970
7. National Institute of Allergy and Infectious Diseases (NIAID)—Est. 1948
8. National Institute of Arthritis and Musculoskeletal and Skin Diseases (NIAMS)—Est. 1986
9. National Institute of Biomedical Imaging and Bioengineering (NIBIB)—Est. 2000
10. Eunice Kennedy Shriver National Institute of Child Health and Human Development (NICHD)—Est. 1962
11. National Institute on Deafness and Other Communication Disorders (NIDCD)—Est. 1988
12. National Institute of Dental and Craniofacial Research (NIDCR)—Est. 1948
13. National Institute of Diabetes and Digestive and Kidney Diseases (NIDDK)—Est. 1950
14. National Institute on Drug Abuse (NIDA)—Est. 1974
15. National Institute of Environmental Health Sciences (NIEHS)—Est. 1969
16. National Institute of General Medical Sciences (NIGMS)—Est. 1962
17. National Institute of Mental Health (NIMH)—Est. 1949
18. National Institute on Minority Health and Health Disparities (NIMHD)—Est. 2010
19. National Institute of Neurological Disorders and Stroke (NINDS)—Est. 1950
20. National Institute of Nursing Research (NINR)—Est. 1986
21. National Library of Medicine (NLM)—Est. 1956
22. NIH Clinical Center (CC)—Est. 1953
23. Center for Information Technology (CIT)—Est. 1964
24. Center for Scientific Review (CSR)—Est. 1946
25. Fogarty International Center (FIC)—Est. 1968
26. National Center for Advancing Translational Sciences (NCATS)—Est. 2011
27. National Center for Complementary and Integrative Health (NCCIH)—Est. 1999

Types of fund based on carrier level (Figs. 8.1 and 8.2; Table 8.1)

Applying for a grant (Fig. 8.3)

Find funding opportunity

- Search http://www.grant.gov for the appropriate funding agency.
- Go to the website of each funding agency to search for specific funding announcements.
- Find the appropriate Study section.
- Contact the Program Official if needed.

Award types

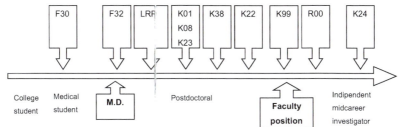

Career stages

FIGURE 8.1   Award type based on career stage.

Award types

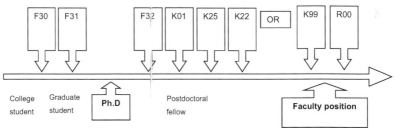

Career stages

FIGURE 8.2   Award type based on career stage.

- Search for other funding opportunities (private, nonprofit foundations, professional organizations, departmental funding etc)

Identify your position
- **Senior faculty/advanced researcher**: Track record of research is important. It should demonstrate strong interest in one topic and that current research is built on the previous research findings.
- **Junior Faculty**/new investigator: Determine whether you qualify as a new investigator. Reviewers will give greater consideration to the proposed approach, rather than the track record for new investigators.

Plan your application
- Review application forms and requirements.
- Look for institutional support and available expertise.
- Contact and communicate with experts who wrote grant applications before.
- Research other resources that can help writing a grant application. (online course, institutional grant writing help course)

TABLE 8.1 Types of funds.

R01	NIH Research Project Grant Program (R01) Used to support a discrete, specified, circumscribed research project NIH's most commonly used grant program No specific dollar limit unless specified in FOA Advance permission required for $500K or more (direct costs) in any year Generally awarded for 3–5 years
R03	NIH Small Grant Program (R03) Provides limited funding for a short period of time to support a variety of types of projects, including: pilot or feasibility studies, collection of preliminary data, secondary analysis of existing data, small, self-contained research projects, development of new research technology, etc. Limited to 2 years of funding Direct costs generally up to $50,000 per year Not renewable Utilized by more than half of the NIH ICs
R13	NIH Support for Conferences and Scientific Meetings (R13 and U13) Support for high quality conferences/scientific meetings that are relevant to NIH's scientific mission and to the public health Requires advance permission from the funding IC Foreign institutions are not eligible to apply Award amounts vary and limits are set by individual ICs Support for up to 5 years may be possible
R15	NIH Academic Research Enhancement Award (AREA) Support small research projects in the biomedical and behavioral sciences conducted by undergraduate and/or graduate students and faculty in institutions of higher education that have not been major recipients of NIH research grant funds Eligibility limited (see https://grants.nih.gov//grants/funding/area.htm) Direct cost limited to $300,000 over entire project period Project period limited to up to 3 years All NIH ICs utilize except FIC and NCATS
R21	NIH Exploratory/Developmental Research Grant Award (R21) Encourages new, exploratory and developmental research projects by providing support for the early stages of project development. Sometimes used for pilot and feasibility studies. Limited to up to 2 years of funding Combined budget for direct costs for the 2 years project period usually may not exceed $275,000. No preliminary data is generally required Most ICs utilize
R34	NIH Clinical Trial Planning Grant (R34) Program Designed to permit early peer review of the rationale for the proposed clinical trial and support development of essential elements of a clinical trial Usually project period of 1 year, sometimes up to 3 Usually, allows for a budget of up to $100,000 direct costs, sometimes up to $450,000 Used only by select ICs; no parent FOA

(Continued)

TABLE 8.1 (Continued)

R41/R42	Small Business Technology Transfer (STTR)
	Intended to stimulate scientific and technological innovation through cooperative research/research and development (R/R&D) carried out between small business concerns (SBCs) and research institutions (RIs)
	Fosters technology transfer between SBCs and RIs
	Assists the small business and research communities in commercializing innovative technologies
	Three-phase structure:
	   1. Feasibility study to establish scientific/technical merit of the proposed R/R&D efforts (generally, 1 year; $150,000)
	   2. Full R/R&D efforts initiated in Phase I (generally 2 years; $1,000,000)
	   3. Commercialization stage (cannot use STTR funds)
	Eligibility limited to United States small business concerns
	Project Director/Principal investigator (PD/PI) may be employed with the SBC *or* the participating nonprofit research institution as long as he/she has a formal appointment with or commitment to the applicant SBC.
	Multiple PD/PIs allowed
	All ICs 🗺 utilize except FIC

R43/R44	Small Business Innovative Research (SBIR)
	Intended to stimulate technological innovation in the private sector by supporting research or research and development (R/R&D) for for-profit institutions for ideas that have potential for commercialization
	Assists the small business research community in commercializing innovative technologies
	Three-phase structure:
	   1. Feasibility study to establish scientific/technical merit of the proposed R/R&D efforts (generally, 6 months; $150,000)
	   2. Full research or R&D efforts initiated in Phase I (generally 2 years; $1,000,000)
	   3. Commercialization stage (cannot use SBIR funds)
	Eligibility limited to United States small business concerns
	The primary employment of the Project Director/Principal investigator (PD/PI) must be with the small business concern.
	Multiple PD/PIs allowed.
	All ICs 🗺 utilize except FIC

R56	NIH High Priority, Short-Term Project Award (R56) Will fund, for 1 or 2 years, high-priority new or competing renewal R01 applications with priority scores or percentiles that fall just outside the funding limits of participating NIH Institutes and Centers (IC). Investigators may not apply for R56 grants.

(*Continued*)

TABLE 8.1 (Continued)

U01	Research Project Cooperative Agreement Supports discrete, specified, circumscribed projects to be performed by investigator(s) in an area representing their specific interests and competencies Used when substantial programmatic involvement is anticipated between the awarding Institute and Center One of many types of cooperative agreements No specific dollar limit unless specified in FOA

K99/R00	NIH Pathway to Independence (PI) Award (K99/R00)
	Also see, New Investigators Program web page
	Provides up to 5 years of support consisting of two phases
	    1. will provide 1−2 years of mentored support for highly promising, postdoctoral research scientists
	    2. up to 3 years of independent support contingent on securing an independent research position
	Award recipients will be expected to compete successfully for independent R01 support from the NIH during the career transition award period
	Eligible Principal Investigators include outstanding postdoctoral candidates who have terminal clinical or research doctorates who have no more than 4 years of postdoctoral research training
	Foreign institutions are not eligible to apply
	PI does not have to be a United States citizen

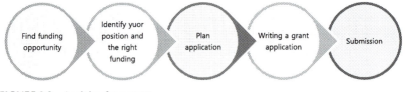

FIGURE 8.3 Applying for a grant.

Summary of federal grants

- A grant is a way the government funds your ideas and projects to provide public services and stimulate the economy. Grants support critical recovery initiatives, innovative research, and many other programs.

Grant lifecycle	
Pre-award phase	Funding opportunity announcement & application review
Award phase	Award decisions & notifications
Post-award phase	Implementation, reporting & closeout

https://www.grants.gov/web/grants/learn-grants/grants-101

Appling for a funding is time consuming

- Finding reliable, substantial scientific research funding is time-consuming, frustrating, and somewhat restrictive to scientific progress.
- University faculty members spent 40% of their research time simply tracking down, writing, and submitting research grant applications. That means that nearly half of the time faculty members using the time for funding instead of actually using their funding and time for research.
- However, without proper funding research cannot be advanced and faculty members are required to obtain funding.
- Less than 20% of the applications for scientific research funding were successfully approved in 2015 according to the National Institutes of Health, meaning that more than 80% of the scientific research applications are rejected.

Writing a grant application

- Review application forms and requirements.
- Look for institutional support and available expertise.
- Contact and communicate with experts who wrote grant applications before.
- Research other resources that can help writing a grant application. (online course, institutional grant writing help course)

Writing a mentoring plan

- Specific mentoring related course detail needs to be demonstrated and documented. The mentoring plan is to demonstrate that research is filling the knowledge gap that exist.
- e.g., Weekly course for platelet receptor function at 7:00 a.m. in the main conference room 503 in Gibbon building.
- Mentoring letters are required that demonstrate adequate mentoring plan for the applicant from several experts in the field.
- The mentor letter needs to match carrier development plan of the applicant (exactly the same course, training that are proposed)

Research plan

- The research plan describes the proposed research, stating its significance and how it will be conducted. The application has two audiences: the majority of reviewers who will probably not be familiar with your topic or field and a smaller number who will be familiar.
- All reviewers are important because each reviewer gets one vote.
  - To succeed in peer review, you must win over the assigned reviewers. They act as your advocates in guiding the review panel's discussion of your application.
  - Write and organize your application so the primary reviewer can readily grasp and explain what you are proposing and advocate for your application.

- Appeal to the reviewers and the funding agency by using language that emphasizes the significance of your proposed work.

Based on NIH grant application the research plan has two sections
1. **Specific aims**—an one-page statement of your objectives for the project.
2. **Research strategy**—a description of the rationale for your research and your experiments in 12 pages for an R01.

Specific aims
- In the specific aims, demonstrate the significance and innovation of your research; then list your two to three concrete objectives, the aims.

Research strategy
- Your research strategy is the key of the application. In this section describe the research rationale and the experiments that will be conducted to accomplish each aim. NIH recommends following these guidelines.
- Organize using bold headers or an outline or numbering system—or both—that you use consistently throughout.
- Start each section with the appropriate header: Significance, Innovation, or Approach.
- Organize the Approach section around your Specific Aims.

Components of research strategy

Significance
- How does the project address an important problem or a critical barrier to progress in the field? If the aims of the project are achieved, how will scientific knowledge, technical capability, and/or clinical practice be improved? How will successful completion of the aims change the concepts, methods, technologies, treatments, services, or preventative interventions that may drive this field and lead to extramural grant funding?

Innovation
- Does the application challenge and seek to shift current research or clinical practice paradigms by utilizing novel theoretical concepts, approaches or methodologies, instrumentation, or interventions? Are these novel to one field of research or in a broader sense?

Approach
- Present a well-reasoned strategy with a brief methodology section that gives confidence in the proposed approach and discuss how the

approach will accomplish the specific aims of the project. Include potential problems to achieving the goals of the project and what benchmarks will be used to determine success. The strategy must address feasibility with the 1 year timeframe and thus the ability to recruit subjects for the study.

Expected outcomes
- Specify expected scientific outcomes.

Statistical analysis & power analysis
- Describe how data will be analyzed. Provide a power calculation that estimates the number of subjects required to demonstrate statistical significance (or an acceptable trend that would justify further pursuit), for data with specific mean group differences and variance, for each outcome.

Innovation & significance
- Innovation and significance are probably the most important section in grant application.
- It needs to demonstrate scientific significance and gap in knowledge.
- It needs to demonstrate both the basic science application and clinical application (e.g., will advance both the field of platelet receptor biology and development of new drugs for platelet inhibitors)
- It needs to demonstrate innovation in concept and approach.

Budget

This step will can be an extremely time-consuming in the writing process.

- Know what type of budget will be required to submit with your application
- Understand the various components of the budget, working with your institution's central grants office and department administrator.
- Contact NIH program officials regarding allowability and other budgetary questions.

Biosketch
- Prepare your biosketch
- Ask for the biosketch from each principal investigator.
- Biosketches are required in both competing applications and progress reports.

- Find instructions, blank format pages, and sample biosketches at: https://grants.nih.gov/grants/forms/biosketch.htm

NIH biographical sketch sample.

BIOGRAPHICAL SKETCH

Provide the following information for the Senior/key personnel and other significant contributors.
Follow this format for each person. **DO NOT EXCEED FIVE PAGES.**

NAME:

eRA COMMONS USER NAME (credential, e.g., agency login):

POSITION TITLE:

EDUCATION/TRAINING **(Begin with baccalaureate or other initial professional education, such as nursing, include postdoctoral training and residency training if applicable. Add/delete rows as necessary.)**

INSTITUTION AND LOCATION	DEGREE (if applicable)	Start Date MM/YYYY	Completion Date MM/YYYY	FIELD OF STUDY

A. Personal Statement

B. Positions and Honors

C. Contributions to Science

D. Additional Information: Research Support and/or Scholastic Performance

YEAR	COURSE TITLE	GRADE

Important writing tips

Make your project's goals realistic

- Be realistic. Do not propose more work than can be reasonably done during the proposed project period. Make sure that the personnel have appropriate scientific expertise and training. Make sure that the budget is reasonable and well-justified.

Be organized and logical
- Start with an outline, following the suggested organization of the application. The thought process of the application should be easy to follow.

Write in clear concise language
- Write a clear topic sentence for each paragraph with one main point or idea. This is key for readability.
- Make your points as direct as possible. Avoid jargon or excessive language.
- Write simple and clear sentences, keeping to about 20 words or less in each.
- Be consistent with terms, references, and writing style.

Sell your idea on paper
- Include enough background information to enable an intelligent reader to understand your proposed work.
- Support your idea with collaborators who have expertise that benefits the project.

Edit yourself, but also enlist help
- Have zero tolerance for typographical errors, misspellings, grammatical mistakes or sloppy formatting. A sloppy or disorganized application may lead the reviewers to conclude that your research may be conducted in the same manner.

Share for comments
- Request your colleagues or mentors review a first draft of your specific aims early in the process. This step can save lots of valuable time.
- Allow time for an internal review by collaborators, colleagues, mentors and make revisions/edits from that review. If possible, have both experts in your field and those who are less familiar with your science provide feedback.

Chapter 9

Data collection

Chapter outline

Data collection

- Data collection is the process of gathering and measuring information on variables of interest, in an established systematic fashion that enables one to answer stated research questions, test hypotheses, and evaluate outcomes. Accurate data collection is essential to maintaining the integrity of research. Both the selection of appropriate data collection instruments (existing, modified, or newly developed) and clearly delineated instructions for their correct use is essential.

Main question for data collection
- Why should something be observed?
- What should be observed?
- How should something be observed?

Methods of data collection
- Biometric measurement
- Questionnaire
- Interview in person
- Phone interview

Biometric measurements
- Biometric measurements are characteristics such as height, weight, body mass index, blood pressure, blood cholesterol, blood glucose, or any other laboratory parameters.
- Biometric measurements can be collected before and after the study intervention to evaluate the effect of the study intervention.

The Practical Guide to Clinical Research and Publication.
DOI: https://doi.org/10.1016/B978-0-12-824517-0.00015-0

Questionnaire

- A questionnaire is a common instrument for data collection.
- It is easier to examine a large number of people with a questionnaire than an in person interview.

Questionnaire databases

- Using existing, validated questionnaires is strongly recommended (Table 9.1).
- Developing a validated questionnaire for a specific research question and data collection is a major project on its own.
- Even already validated questionnaires must be checked if it is suitable for the study population and the specific research question.

TABLE 9.1 Questionnaire database.

Questionnaire databases
Economic and social research council survey question bank (UK) https://www.ukdataservice.ac.uk/
CDC national health interviews surveys (USA) https://www.cdc.gov/nchs/nhis/nhis_questionnaires.htm

Developing a questionnaire

- A newly developed questionnaire must be validated to meet the standards of epidemiological research and evidence-based medicine.
- The effort involved in developing a questionnaire should not be underestimated.
- It is easier and time saving to use a questionnaire that has been already validated.
- A validated questionnaire is not always available to the specific research question.

The following should be defined first before implementing a questionnaire:

- Is it a quantitative or qualitative data collection?
- Type of survey: is it a phone interview, in person interview, email survey?
- Questionnaire size: questionnaires that are too long will not be completed.
- Sample size: how many samples do I need to answer the research question?
- Population/target group: it is difficult to collect data from children or elderly using a questionnaire.
- Survey period: avoid seasonal bias.

- Survey location: avoid geographical or location related bias.
- How will the survey be implemented?
- Define primary outcome.
- Define secondary outcome.
- Data recruitment.
- Data cleanup: how do I deal with unanswered questions or duplicated answers?
- Statistical analysis: which statistical analytical method will be used?
- How should the questionnaire be designed in order to be able to code it afterwards for statistical analysis?

Open-ended questions
What is your age? _____ Years
What is your nationality? _____
Closed-ended question (yes/no questions)
Do you use internet? □ yes □ no
Categorical questions
What is your marital status? □ single □ married □ divorced □ widowed
Rating scales

	Always	Often	Sometimes	Rarely	Never
I found the waiting time from admission to treatment too long	[0]	[1]	[2]	[3]	[4]

Examples of poor questions

1. How did doctors and nursing staff responded to the new 45-minute lunch break?
   □ Satisfied
   □ Unsatisfied
   Split double questions.
   □ *How did doctors react to the new 45-minute lunch break?*
   □ *How did nursing staff react to the new 45-minute lunch break?*
2. Do you think smoking in pregnancy is dangerous for mother and child?
   Split double questions.
   □ *Do you think smoking in pregnancy is dangerous for the mother?*
   □ *Do you think smoking in pregnancy is dangerous for the child?*
3. What is your monthly household income?
   □ < 1000 €
   □ 1000−2000 €

☐ 2000–3000 €

☐ > € 3000

Avoid overlapping numbers.

☐ *1000–1999*

☐ *2000–2999*

4. Which newspaper do you read?

Formulate a question very specifically

☐ *How many newspapers do you read?*

☐ *Which newspaper have you read in the last month (multiple selection)*

☐ *Did you change the newspaper last month?*

5. Do you have a tooth with amalgam filling?

☐ Yes

☐ No

Offer enough options!

Consider the option "others" or "free text" as an answer choice.

Checklist to review a questionnaire

Things that should be considered during developing a questionnaire

- Is the first question given special attention?
- Are the subject areas and the order of the questions appropriate?
- Have difficult or sensitive questions been well thought out and formulated?
- Is there an "other" or "free text" category?
- Are there any filter questions?
- Is the layout appropriate (format, step size, paper quality)?
- Is the layout of responses appropriate? (Uniform)

Things to clarify before implementing the questionnaire

- Who is conducting the survey?
- Who is responsible, who can the study patient contact in case there is a question?
- What is the purpose or goal of the research?
- What is the study population?
- What happens to the questionnaire results?
- Will the questionnaire results be available to the public?
- How much time needs to be invested?

Important

- Every question in the questionnaire should be answered
- Avoid multiple selection possibilities unless it is truly indicated.

- Simplify answer options of each question. Statistical analysis will be easier with simplified coding.
- Consider all people who are involved in the project when creating a questionnaire (researchers, interviewers, respondents, data managers, and statisticians)
- Make questions short, simple and clear
- Ask specific questions in a neutral way. Avoid terms like "better," "healthier" etc.
- Pretest! Pretest! Pretest! Pretest! Pretest the questionnaire and modify it before implementing it.

Pilot phase
- Test the questionnaire on multiple people, because not everyone interprets the same question the same way.
- Test the questionnaire several times in different groups and individuals
- A pretest is carried out and checked according to the Beywl/Schepp-Winter criteria (possibly another pretest)
- This optimizes questions and answers
- Remove ambiguities in questions and answers
- Estimate time expenditure

Questionnaire review (Beywl/Schepp-Winter 2000)
- Are there any unnecessary questions?
- Are all questions easy to understand?
- Can the respondents answer the questions in a meaningful way?
- Can the respondents understand the instructions?
- Does the questionnaire contain abbreviations, technical terms, and colloquial expressions that may not be understood by everyone?
- Is the number of response categories large enough so that differentiations are possible/small enough so that not in the evaluation?
- Several answer categories remain empty?
- Is the arch structured logically?
- Can introductions, transitions, ... be read fluently?
- Does the questionnaire keep the respondents interested?

Evaluation after data collection
- If possible, the survey response rate should always be calculated and reported.
- It should be discussed how to handle missing data.

Bias in data collection using a questionnaire
- Not all questions in the questionnaire are understood correctly.
- Language can be act as a barrier.

- Skipping answers is common phenomenon.
- "Socially undesirable" actions are not answered truthfully (e.g., alcoholics, smokers tend to indicate lower consumption).
- Drug use or sex behavior related questions are often not answered (fear/embarrassment).

Example
Questionnaire—Research question: Social inequality in health care.

Example of a questionnaire development
    Social inequality in health care
    Hypothesis: Lower socioeconomic status patients are treated inferiorly in the emergency department at night than the socially higher ones (in Berlin).
    Quantitative data collection
    Type of survey: Written survey in the form of a questionnaire.
    Questionnaire scope: four pages with 12 questions (social class assessment), 21 questions (health care assessment).
    Pretest: A pretest is carried out and reviewed according to the criteria of Beywl/Schepp-Winter (2000) (possibly another pretest is performed)
    Sample size: $n =$ consultation with the statistician.
    Population: All (over 18 years) who come to the hospital for treatment (including those who leave the hospital without treatment).
    (No intensive care patients because in most cases the maximum medial care is performed and the patients are usually not able to answer questionnaires)
    Survey period: May 1, 2020–May 1, 2021 to avoid any seasonal differences.
    Location: All hospitals with an emergency room in Berlin.
    Implementation: Written survey with questionnaire.
    (Two pages on the social class, two pages on health care).
    Process: The questionnaire should be completed while waiting for the discharge letter If an inpatient admission takes place, the questionnaire will be filled out the following day. Patients who leave the hospital without treatment will get the questionnaire with a stamped envelope when they sign "leave against medical advice."
    Primary outcome: Satisfaction, waiting time, and doctor-patient relationship
    Secondary outcome: Demographics of patients in the emergency room (age, social class, and nationality).
    Data recruitment: Reminders of the hospital at different time intervals.
    Data cleansing: Review questionnaires that are not properly filled out and have missing information and sort them out if necessary.
    Statistical evaluation: SAS, SPSS

Research question

The night shift poses a special challenge for everyone, including experienced doctors or medical staff. Insufficient staffing during night shift, makes it difficult for doctors or nurses to treat patients quickly and satisfactorily. Long waiting times and limited treatments are not uncommon, especially in the emergency room at night (night shift is defined as the time from 8:00 p.m. to the next day at 8:00 a.m.). The question arises whether there are differences in care depending on the social class of the patient.

Goal setting

The objective of the study is to clarify whether social layer-based disparities exist in patient care in the emergency room at night.

Hypothesis

Socially weaker patients are treated inferiorly in the emergency department at night than the socially stronger ones.

Operationalization of the central concepts

Subjects characteristics

- Age: the age is queried as free text. This can subsequently be represented as an ordinal scaling in age groups if necessary.
- Gender: binary scaling
- Nationality: free text
- Marital status: nominally scaled
- Insurance status: nominally scaled

Social class

"Social class" is a term that "denotes a category of members of society who have common characteristics with regard to vertical social structure or social inequality: in particular the same or similar socioeconomic situation (position in professional life, income and wealth situation), life chances and social recognition of social prestige" (Hillman 1994).

The social class index according to Winkler has proven to be a useful tool to evaluate and categorize the social classes among individuals. It expresses the complexity in social differentiation in consideration of various factors including: income, professional position and education (J Wrappers 1999 Winkler J 1998).

Likewise, according to the DAE recommendation (German Working Group on Epidemiology), the social class is made up of income, education and professional position. In addition to these characteristics, some authors include other indicators of social classes. However since there is disagreement among these characteristics, it is recommended by the DAE to limit social class characteristics to the three aspects mentioned (Jöckel KH 1998).

Education

Here you are asked for the highest degree. The categorization of "education" is not easy due to the different education systems in different countries. In order to make a compromise between the detail and the length, it was queried in the following six categories:

- no graduation
- Professional school

(Continued)

(Continued)

- *High school graduation*
- *Bachelor*
- *Master*
- *Doctorate*

Professional status position
Due to the complexity of the professional status clear distinction is difficult. The professional status position is categorized in nine items: Self-employed, in training, unskilled/semiskilled workers, skilled workers, government employee, academics, top position (CEO)/professors, no information.

Net household income
The household net income was, collected in a two-step query as recommended by the DAE. The first question openly asked about the income amount. In a second step, those who do not want to or cannot specify the exact amount of income had the option to check a box from a list of income classes.

However, since many income earners do not have their own income but share it with the other people in the household, the additional determination of the household size and the age of the household members is required to determine the equalized income.

Hospital care
Documenting "patient care" in the hospital setting in order to analyze it later is challenging. Several different characteristics are used to document "patient care" accurately.
- *Doctor-patient relationship (trust in doctor, doctor behavior, sufficient information, participation in decisions, communication)*
- *Waiting times for treatment*
- *Duration of the doctors interview*
- *The request to visit the doctor was fulfilled*
- *Improvement in health since treatment*
- *Personal feelings*
- *etc.*

Consideration in the survey
Since the socially weaker group must be given special consideration in the documentation, the scaling is carried out uniformly ordinal in five categories "not at all" to "is completely correct." Also, due to possible language barriers, only few open questions are included.

Questionnaire
One page introduction, two pages social characteristics, two pages patient care.

Questionnaire
Emergency room patient care at night

Dear patient!

The questionnaire is designed to evaluate your experience during the emergency room treatment. For better understanding and to answer the questions apporiately, you will find some **explanations and examples below** :

Please check only **one** answer at a time, the one that best suits your experience.

Example: "The support was satisfactory."

Not true   Rarely true   Somewhat true   Mostly true
Completely true
[0] [1] [2] [3] [4]

Please complete the questionnaire by checking the appropriate box.

Example: "How were you admitted to the hospital?"
Emergency admission   planned admission
[]   []

When necessary, please enter a number or free text.

Example: "What is your age?" .... years

Please answer **all** questions and statements as carefully as possible!
All information in this interview is being kept confidential.

If you have any questions , please contact Dr. Y
Tel: 030 000 001

Date: day / month / year v1	time v1-1	
What is your age? years v2		
What is your gender?	[] male v3 [] female v3	
What is your nationality?	v4	
What marital status do you have? V5	[] single v5-1 [] married v5-2 [] divorced v5-3 [] widowed v5-4	
What is your insured status? V6	[] without insurance v6-1 [] government insured v6-2] *with additional insurance v6-2-1* [] privately insured v6-3	
What is your highest achieved Graduation? V7	[] without graduation v7-1 [] professional school v7-2 [] high school v7-3 [] bachelor v7-4 [] master v7-5 [] doctorate v7-6	
What professional position do you have? V8	[] independent v8-1 [] in training v8-2 [] Un- / semi-skilled v8-4 [] Skilled workers v8-5 [] Employees v8-6 [] Government employee v8-7 [] Academics v8-8 [] top position (CEO) / Professor v8-9 [] not specified v8-10	
What is your monthly net income? v10	Euro v10-1 [] no income v10-2 [] not specified v10-3	
Which letter from this list here applies to your net income? V11-1 to V11-20		

B	Under € 300	S	4,000 to less than 4,500€
T	300 to less than 600 €	K	4,500 to under 5,000 €
P	600 to less than € 1,000€	O	5,000 to less than 5,500 €
F	1,000 to less than 1,400 €	C.	5 500 to less than 6 000€
E	1,400 to less than 1,800€	G	6,000 to less than € 6,500€
H	1,800 to less than 2,200 €	U	6,500 to less than 7,000 €
L	2,200 to less than 2,500 €	J	7,000 to under 7,500 €
N	2,500 to less than 3,000 €	V	7,500 to under 10,000 €
R	3,000 to less than 3,500 €	Q	10,000 to under 15,000 €
M	3 500 to less than 4 000 €	W	15,000 €and more

What is the total monthly net income of your **household?** v12	Euro v12-1 [] no income v12-2 [] not specified v12-3
Which letter from this list here applies to your household's net income? V13-1 to V13-20	
How many people in your household are 18 or older?	v14

Patient care

What was the reason for the emergency room? V15	[] Accident v15-1
	[] Sudden complaints v15-2 [] Heart v15-2-1 [] Gastrointestinal v15-2-2 [] Kidney v15-2-3 [] Back (upper) v15-2-4 [] Extremities (arms, legs) v15-2-5 [] Back (lower) v15-3 [] Head v15-4

	Not true	Rarely true	Somewhat true	Mostly true	Completely true
I felt the waiting time from the admission until treatment as too long. v16	[0]	[1]	[2]	[3]	[4]
Even before the doctor's was able to see me, I was treated for my symptoms. v17	[0]	[1]	[2]	[3]	[4]
The staff always responded helpful to my pain and complaints. v18	[0]	[1]	[2]	[3]	[4]
The medical staff looked overly stressed, tired or irritated. v19	[0]	[1]	[2]	[3]	[4]
The doctors were always available for any problems. v20	[0]	[1]	[2]	[3]	[4]
The treating doctors were kind to me. v21	[0]	[1]	[2]	[3]	[4]
The doctor carried out the necessary medical measures safely and thoroughly. v21	[0]	[1]	[2]	[3]	[4]
It bothered me that the medical examination was carried out in the presence of strangers. v22	[0]	[1]	[2]	[3]	[4]
The amount of time, that the doctor was available was too short. v23	[0]	[1]	[2]	[3]	[4]

(Continued)

(Continued)

	Not true	Rarely true	Somewhat true	Mostly true	Completely true
The waiting times between the examinations were too long. v24	[0]	[1]	[2]	[3]	[4]
I was notified and thoroughly explained about the interim results of my medical exam/lab values or imaging's. v25	[0]	[1]	[2]	[3]	[4]
The doctor answered all my open questions. v26	[0]	[1]	[2]	[3]	[4]
The nature and cause of my illness/disease is still unclear to me. v27	[0]	[1]	[2]	[3]	[4]
The doctors gave me the recommendation to return if new symptoms or complications occur. v28	[0]	[1]	[2]	[3]	[4]
The overall doctors visit was satisfactory. v29	[0]	[1]	[2]	[3]	[4]
I have the feeling that the doctor did not take my complaints seriously. v30	[0]	[1]	[2]	[3]	[4]
I have the feeling that the doctor did not carry out the necessary treatment despite the need. v31	[0]	[1]	[2]	[3]	[4]
I feel better after the treatment. v32	[0]	[1]	[2]	[3]	[4]
The overall treatment was satisfactory. v33	[0]	[1]	[2]	[3]	[4]
I would return to the same hospital in the future, in the event of an emergency. v34	[0]	[1]	[2]	[3]	[4]

*All encodings from v16 to v34 have the subcoding v (X) −1 to v (X) −5.

How do you rate your overall hospital stay? v35-1 to v35-10									
Very bad → Excellent									
[0]	[1]	[2]	[3]	[4]	[5]	[6]	[7]	[8]	[9]

Thank you for your cooperation!
V = variable
Each question is then coded with 0, 1 in Excel.

Discussion: evaluation of the strengths and weaknesses of the research approach.

Is the method appropriate?

There are clear advantages and disadvantages of a written survey (Gerl, Herbert/Pehl, Klaus, 1983). The written survey significantly reduces the activity of those involved. There are also systematic failures (people with a higher level of education are more likely to respond than people with a low level of education). It is difficult to evaluate whether the recruited patient filled out the survey him/herself or eventually the accompanying person. The advantages of a written survey is the quick and extensive patient/participant evaluation. It is particularly advantageous for quantitative methods, as is the case here.

Is the method of measuring social class appropriate?

The analysis of the social status according to the recommendations of the GPE consists of the three characteristics income, education and professional position. However, based on the limited length of the questionnaire, it is not possible to follow the full and extensive evaluation method as per recommendation. However, a questionnaire should not exceed a total of 25 units or 10 min (Bosnjak, Michael/Batinic, Bernad, 1999; Gräf and Lorenz, 1999), the length and the survey about the social class are appropriate.

Are the questions about measuring patient care in the emergency room appropriate? (reliability, validity)

What other characteristics can be used to measure the patient care quality?

This question represents the specific challenge in the developing a questionnaire. Since there are no standardized questionnaires for this specific research question, a diverse comparison with other similar questionnaires should be performed. Sufficient pretesting should also be carried out to uncover and improve the shortcomings or incomprehensibility of the questionnaire.

Validation of the questionnaire will not be feasible in this research approach due to the time limit. Alternatively, a face validation can be performed.

Is the questionnaire adequate?

- Is the questionnaire too long?
- Is the questionnaire measuring what should be measured?
- Is it possible to analyze all patients with the same questionnaire?
- Do all criteria apply to all patients?
- Can the weak social classes answer the questionnaire appropriately?
- Are there any difficulties in answering due a language barrier?

Are there any difficulties in the implementation?

A pilot test should be carried out in order to uncover possible existing errors or improvement points. If unexpected difficulties in the implementation of the survey is found, they can be adjusted before implementing the study.

Supplemented by the quantitative method

Different validation methods can be used to achieve higher validity. It is recommended to combine qualitative and quantitative methods in research for better data collection. In this study design, qualitative method was not used.

(Continued)

(Continued)

Conclusion

Overall, this concept is a good approach to answer the research question. However, the review and further development of the questionnaire and repeated testing is necessary. A pilot study should be carried out in order to identify any remaining problems or difficulties in the questionnaire and in the study design and to eliminate them as best as possible.

Quality criteria

Reliability

- Reliability is about the consistency of a measurement (precision) (Fig. 9.1).
- A specific measure is considered to be reliable if its application, on the same object of measurement, number of times produces the same results.

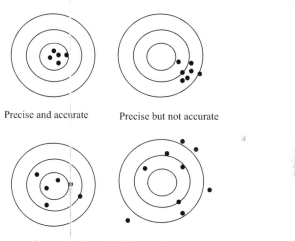

Precise and accurate   Precise but not accurate

Accurate but not precise   Neither precise nor accurate

FIGURE 9.1   Systematic measurement and errors.

Example

A reliable research question is: How many medical students are there in one semester.

A low reliable research question is: How many smart medical students are in one semester.

Reliability test methods
Test-retest correlation

- A test is carried out to the same people twice at different times to see if the scores are the same.

- The reliability of its results is measured based on the discrepancies between the results of the first and second tests.

Parallel testing
- Parallel forms of the test are carried out on the same group of subjects

Split-half reliability testing
- In split-half reliability, a test for a single knowledge area is split into two parts and then both parts given to one group of students at the same time. The scores from both parts of the test are correlated.

Validity
- Validity refers to how accurately a method measures what it is intended to measure.

Example
Trying to measure students "intelligence" based on their shoe size is an example of a nonvalid measurement.

A standardized test results or an IQ test would be a valid measurement for the "intelligence" of the students.

Face validity
- Face validity is simply whether the test appears (at face value) to measure what it claims to.
- Agreement of the measured results with the subjective assessments of experts.
- This is the least sophisticated measure of validity.

Content validity
- Content validity is how well an instrument (i.e., a test or questionnaire) measures a theoretical construct.
- To produce valid results, the content of a test, survey or measurement method must cover all relevant parts of the subject it aims to measure. If some aspects are missing from the measurement (or if irrelevant aspects are included), the validity is threatened.
- Therefore, content validity is the basis of a construct validity.
- The content validity cannot be determined objectively and quantitatively and is therefore assessed by experts and the study investigator.

Criterion validity
- Criterion validity is an estimate of the extent to which a measure agrees with an established standard of comparison (i.e., a criterion).
- Criterion = external criterion (e.g., another test that is gold standard)

Concurrent validity
- The external criterion was collected simultaneously with the measurement

Example
A newly developed psychological test is tested and compared simultaneously with an already validated psychological test.

Predictive validity
- The external criterion is collected after the measurement.

Example
Those students who have good grades at school have a better career in the future.

Construct validity
- Construct validity defines how well a test or experiment measures up to its claims. It refers to whether the operational definition of a variable actually reflect the true theoretical meaning of a concept.
- The survey procedure must be embedded in a theoretical concept and should be consistency with existing theories.

Convergent validity
- Convergent validity takes two measures that are supposed to be measuring the same construct and shows that they are related.

Discriminant validity
- Discriminant validity shows that two measures that are not supposed to be related are in fact, unrelated.

Internal validity
- Internal validity refers to the degree of validity/confidence that the causal relationship being tested is trustworthy and not influenced by other factors or variables.

External validity
- External validity refers to the extent to which results from a study can be applied (generalized) to other situations, groups or events.

Internal validity is the basis for external validity.

Objectivity
- Objectivity is the true finding of the causality of a research independent from the study investigators influence.

Quality of life measuring instruments

Quality adjusted life years = QALY

- The quality-adjusted life year is a measure of the value and benefit of health outcomes.
- Since health is a function of length of life and quality of life, the QALY was developed as an attempt to combine the value of these attributes into a single index number.
- A QALY of 1 means a year in full health, while a QALY of 0 means death.

Disability adjusted life years = DALY

- Disability adjusted life years is the sum of years of potential life lost due to premature mortality and the years of productive life lost due to disability.
- DALY = YLL + YLD
- YLL—*Years lived with disability:* years of life lost through premature death
    - YLL = N × L
    - N = number of deaths
    - L = standard life expectancy at age of death in years
- YLD—*Years of life lost:* years of life lived with disabilities.
    - YLD = I × DW × L
    - I = number of incident cases
    - DW = disability weight
    - L = average duration of the case until remission or death (years)

QALY
Advantage
- Is relatively easy to implement.
- Integration of effects on lifespan and quality.

Disadvantage
- QALY ratings do not necessarily agree with the individual's assessment.
- Systematic influence of the (expected) remaining lifetime.
- For diseases in which the focus of the treatment is not the prolongation of life but the reduction of illness-related impairments or the improvement of quality of life, the determination and interpretation of QALYs is problematic

DALY
Advantage
- DALY can be used to compare different countries.
- DALY is only used at the level of large populations, mostly for addressing issues of international health policy.

- The biggest advantage is that morbidity (YLD) and mortality (YLL) effects are combined in one measure.
- DALY allow the comparison between different health hazards.
- The DALY measure offers the ability to assess the impact of prevention strategies

Disadvantage
- The expected years of life are different in each population and therefore the years of life lost depends on the population that was selected.
- There are differences in the expected years of life for women and men.
- There is no clear answer to who and how is "disability" is defined?

SF-36
- The short form (SF) (36) health survey is a 36-item, patient-reported survey of patient health. The SF-36 is a measure of health status and an abbreviated variant of it, the SF-6D, is commonly used in health economics as a variable in the quality-adjusted life year calculation to determine the cost-effectiveness of a health treatment.

Chapter 10

Scaling and coding

Chapter outline

Scaling and coding

Scaling

- Scales of measurement refer to ways in which variables/numbers are defined and categorized.
- Each scale of measurement has certain properties which in turn determines the appropriateness for use of certain statistical analyses.
- The four scales of measurement are nominal, ordinal, interval, and ratio.
- When using an existing database, it is important to know how the variables are scaled (Fig. 10.1 and Table 10.1).

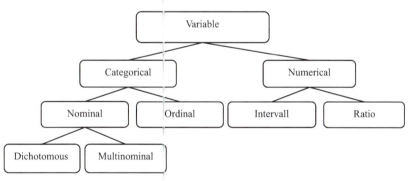

FIGURE 10.1 Variables and its types.

Categories of variables

Ordinal

- An ordinal scale of measurement represents an ordered series of relationships or rank order.
- Ordinal variables can be considered "in between" categorical and quantitative variables.

The Practical Guide to Clinical Research and Publication.
DOI: https://doi.org/10.1016/B978-0-12-824517-0.00003-4

TABLE 10.1 Examples of variables.

Scale level	Examples
Nominal scale	Sex (male/female)
Ordinal scale	Soccer team ranking (rank 1−18)
Interval scale	Temperature (−100°C to 100°C), annual numbers
Ratio scale	Age (0−99 years)
Absolute scale	Population of a country

Example

Score: 1−14

Satisfaction (very satisfied > rather satisfied > rather unsatisfied > very unsatisfied)

Nominal
- A nominal variable has two or more categories, but there is no intrinsic ordering to the categories.
- Categorical data and numbers are simply used as identifiers or names.

Example

Dog = 1. Cat = 2, Mouse = 3

Dichotomous
- A dichotomous variable is one that takes on one of only two possible values when observed or measured.

Example

*The variable "sex" has two forms, male and female. It is therefore a **dichotomous, nominal variable**.*

Continuous variable

Interval
- The interval variable is a measurement variable that is used to define values measured along a scale, with each point placed at an equal distance from one another.
- The value zero represents simply an additional point of measurement in an interval scale.
- The Celsius/Fahrenheit scale is a good example of the interval scale of measurement.

Example

Years, temperature in Celsius/Fahrenheit

Ratio
- The ratio scale of measurement is similar to the interval scale in that it also represents quantity and has equality of units.
- However, this scale also has an absolute zero (no numbers exist below the zero).

Example

Blood pressure, temperature in Kelvin, age.

Coding
- Coding is the process of labeling and organizing your qualitative data to identify different themes and the relationships between them.
- Microsoft Excel is one of the most commonly used encoding software.
- Excel can be imported into many statistical software programs.
- The collated data should be coded largely in the numbers "0" and "1".
- Divide the categories as far as possible and code with "0" and "1".
- Free text needs to be coded into categories or numbers.
- If there is no data available for a certain criteria, leave the field blank. Do not code with "0" since "0" is an information.

Example

Men = 1, Woman = 0 (Table 10.2).
  Received chest x-ray = 1, did not receive chest x-ray = 0.
  CT performed = 1, CT not performed = 0.

No data available = leave the field blank. Missing data
- Human errors are the most common. Review dataset.
- Try to complete the dataset as accurately as possible.
- Inadequate or incorrectly collected data cannot be cleaned up by sophisticated statistical analysis.

If completion of the missing data is not possible several options are available.

1. Accepted that the value is missing, and the statistical analysis is carried out without the value.
2. The subject is excluded from the analysis.
3. Missing data are replaced with mean values.
4. Consult a statistician for different statistical options how to deal with missing values.

TABLE 10.2 Example of coding the collected data into an Excel sheet.

N	Name	Sex	DOB	CXR	CT	CT-head	S100	S100 abnormal	CGS score (3–15)	GCS 13–15	GCS 12–9	GCS <8	Thoracic trauma
1	Smith	1	1958	1	1	1	1.99	1	14	1	0	0	0
2	Meyer	1	1964	1	1	0	0.631	1	15	1	0	0	0
3	Miller	1	1942	1	1	0	0.077	0	15	1	0	0	0
4	Brown	1	1999	1	0	1	5.34	1	11	0	1	0	1
5	McNulen	0	1921	0	0	0	0.049	0	10	0	1	0	0
6	Patel	1	1972	1	1	0	1.37	1	15	1	0	0	1
7	Johnson	1	1954	0	0	0	1.39	1	15	1	0	0	1
8	William	1	1971	1	1	0	0.055	0	12	0	1	0	1
9	Jones	1	1925	1	0	1	9.56	1	8	0	0	1	1
10	Davis	0	1965	1	0	1	1.68	1	15	1	0	0	0
11	Rodriguez	1	1987	1	0	1	1.35	1	15	1	0	0	1
12	Kim	0	1990	1	0	1	4.83	1	7	0	0	1	0
13	Lee	1	1928	1	0	0	0.497	1	15	1	0	0	0
14	Lopez	1	1962	1	0	1	0.205	1	15	1	0	0	0
15	Thomas	0	1942	1	1	0	0.928	1	15	1	0	0	0
1H	Gonzales	1	1935	1	1	1	2.94	1	12	0	1	0	1
17	Moore	0	1952	1	0	1	0.098	0	8	0	0	1	0

S100, Brain tumor marker (protein S100); CXR, chest x-ray; CT, computed tomography; CGS, Glasgow Coma Scale.

Chapter 11

Statistical tests

Chapter outline

Statistic software

- The most commonly used statistical software in biostatistics are SPSS, SAS, and STATA (Table 11.1).

TABLE 11.1 Comparison of SPSS, SAS, STATA.

	SPSS	SAS	STATA
Ease of use	Medium	Medium/difficult	Easy/medium
Analytics properties	Large	Almost unlimited	Large
Data processing	Large	Very large	Medium
Program utilization (CPU)	Medium	Large	Little
Programming	Yes	Yes	Yes
Open source	No	No	Yes
Extensibility	Difficult	Difficult	Easy
Price	Medium	Expensive	Cheap
Homepage	www.ibm.com/ software/ analytics/spss	www.sas.com	www.stata.com

The Practical Guide to Clinical Research and Publication.
DOI: https://doi.org/10.1016/B978-0-12-824517-0.00004-6

Types of statistical tests
- Chi^2 test ($=$chi-square test $= \chi^2$ test)
- Fisher exact test
- Student T-Test (T-Test)
- ANOVA
- Linear regression
- Logistic regression
- Poison regression
- Kaplan Meier curve
- Log-rank test
- Cox regression
- Correlation coefficient
- Cronbach's Alpha
- Cohen's Kappa

Comparison of proportions

Chi-square test

Indication
- The chi-square test is used to calculate the frequency of distribution.
- The chi-square test is used to calculate the independency between two categorical characteristics.
- H_0: proportions in both groups are the same
    = Exposure and outcome are independent.
- H_1: Proportions in both groups are different
    = Exposure and outcome are not independent.

Requirement
- Nominal dichotomous variables.
- Four-field table (2×2 tables) (four-field table = one degree of freedom).
- An adequately large sample size is required for adequate testing (≥ 20).
- An adequately large sample size in each cell is required (> 5).
- A chi-square test can also be performed with 3×3, 4×4 ... table. However, interpretation between the connections of the variables is complex.

Interpretation
- The "critical value" is 3.84 (one degree of freedom, $1 - \alpha = 95\%$).
- If chi-squared test is > 3.84 then the null hypothesis (H_0) is rejected.
- Depending on how large the value is, the statistical software automatically calculates the α-value.
- The α-value can also be obtained manually from the table (Table 11.2).

TABLE 11.2 Quantiles of the chi-square distribution.

f	$1-\alpha$					
	0.900	0.950	0.975	0.990	0.995	0.999
1	2.71	3.84	5.02	6.63	7.88	10.83
2	4.61	5.99	7.38	9.21	10.60	13.82
3	6.25	7.81	9.35	11.34	12.84	16.27
4	7.78	9.49	11.14	13.28	14.86	18.47
5	9.24	11.07	12.83	15.09	16.75	20.52
6	10.64	12.59	14.45	16.81	18.55	22.46
7	12.02	14.07	16.01	18.48	20.28	24.32
8	13.36	15.51	17.53	20.09	21.95	26.12
9	14.68	16.92	19.02	21.67	23.59	27.88
10	15.99	18.31	20.48	23.21	25.19	29.59

f = Degree of freedom, α = level of significance.

Number of degrees of freedom(f) = Number of rows $-$ 1 $\cdot$ number of columns $-$ 1

Limitations
- If the sample size is too small the chi-square test cannot be used (use Fischer exact test instead).

Example

	Variable 1	Variable 2	Variable 3	Variable 4	Variable 5
Patient	Gender	Hypertension	Heart attack		
1	1	0	1		
2	0	1	1		
3	0	1	0		
4	1	0	0		
5	1	0	1		
6	0	1	1		
7	1	0	0		
.	.	.	.		
.	.	.	.		

1 = yes, 0 = no (sex: 1 = man, 0 = woman)
Hypothesis: Men have heart attacks more often than women.
Chi-square test: Compare variable 1 with variable 3

$\chi^2 = 10.8 \; 10 > 3.84 \; H_0$: *reject P = .001*
→ *Men have heart attack more often than women.*
$\chi^2 = 2.7 \; 10 < 3.84 \; H_1$: *do not reject P = .1*
→ *Men don't have heart attacks more often than women.*

Fisher exact test
- *If the number of cases in a single cell is <5, or the total number of cases is <20, the use of Fischer Exakt Test is more appropriate.*
- *In SPSS, the Fischer test can be included in the chi-square test. (simply read the value from the analysis table).*

Comparison of mean values

Assumption for a statistical test
- The population must be close to a normal distribution.
- Samples must be independent.
- Population variances must be equal.
- Groups must have equal sample sizes.

Data distribution
- The distribution of date should be analyzed first, since different statistical tests are used based on the distribution of the values (Fig. 11.1).

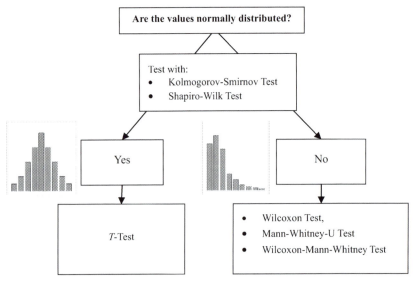

FIGURE 11.1 Distribution of values.

- The distribution of the data can be checked with the Kolmogorov-Smirnov test or Shapiro-Wilk test.
- If the data is normally distributed, a T-Test can be used.

If the data follows an abnormal distribution a nonparametric test should be used:

- Wilcoxon test.
- Mann-Whitney U-test.
- Wilcoxon-Mann-Whitney Test.
- With a large number of cases (>30 per group), the T-Test can also be used.

One-sample T-Test (Student's T-Test)
- A T-Test is used to determine if there is a significant difference between the means of two groups.
- The one-sample T-Test is a statistical hypothesis test used to determine whether an unknown population mean is different from a predetermined specific value.

Example

- *Do I normally get by with €500 a month?*
- *Does the cafeteria meal cost an average of €2.50?*
- *Is my cars average gas mileage 24 mpg?*

T-Test for two independent samples
- The independent samples T-Test compares the means of two independent groups in order to determine whether there is statistical evidence that the associated population means are significantly different.
- The independent Samples T-Test is a parametric test.
- The independent T-Test is also known as unpaired T-Test.
- The group can be formed using a dichotomous (0, 1) variable (e.g., male = 1, female = 0)
- The primary assumption of all comparative tests is always "there is no statistical difference between the two independent groups"
- For ordinal scaled variables Mann-Whitney U-test, Kolmogorov-Smirnov test, etc. are used.
  - H_0: mean values in both groups are not different
  - H_1: mean values in the two groups are different

Example

Patient	Variable 1 Sex	Variable 2 Drug	Variable 3 Hypertension	Variable 4 Heart attack	Variable 5 Systolic blood pressure
1	1	1	0	1	120
2	0	1	1	1	155
3	0	1	1	0	143
4	1	1	0	0	129
5	1	0	0	1	131
6	0	0	1	1	160
7	1	0	0	0	130
.	.	.	.		
.	.	.	.		

1 = yes, 0 = no (sex: 1 = man, 0 = woman)

Hypothesis: Men have increased systolic pressure more often than women.

T-Test: comparing variable 1 with variable 5

Dependent *T*-Test (paired *T*-Test)
- The dependent *T*-Test (also called the paired *T*-Test or paired-samples *T*-Test) compares the means of two related groups to determine whether there is a statistically significant difference between these means.
- A paired *T*-Test simply calculates the difference between paired observations (e.g., before and after) and then performs a one-sample *T*-Test on the differences.
- It tests whether the mean difference in the pairs (two sets of observation) is different from zero.

Exampleot

Patient	Variable 1 Gender	Variable 2 Hypertension	Variable 3 Drug A	Variable 4 Systolic blood pressure before therapy	Variable 5 Systolic blood pressure after therapy
1	1	0	1	140	130
2	0	1	0	155	150
3	0	1	0	145	150
4	1	0	1	160	150
5	1	0	1	145	140
6	0	1	0	155	155
7	1	0	1	150	145
.	.	.	.		
.	.	.	.		

1 = yes, 0 = no (sex: 1 = man, 0 = woman)
Hypothesis: Drug A lowers blood pressure.
T-Test: Compare variable 3 with variable 4 and variable 5.

ANOVA (analysis of variance)

- The analysis of variance (ANOVA) is used to determine whether there are any statistically significant differences between the means of two or more independent (unrelated) variables/groups.
- The null hypothesis for the test is that the two means are equal. Therefore, a significant result means that the two means are unequal.
- A one way ANOVA will tell you that at least two groups were different from each other. But it won't tell you which groups were different. If your test returns a significant f-statistic, you may need to run an ad hoc test (like the Least Significant Difference test) to tell you exactly which groups had a difference in means.

Example

Testing the relationship between weight loss and drinks: coffee, soda, black tea, and green tea.

Two way ANOVA

- With a one way, there is one independent variable affecting a dependent variable.
- With a two way ANOVA, there are two independent variables affecting a dependent variable.
- The only difference between one-way and two-way ANOVA is the number of independent variables.

Example

Testing the relationship between weight loss and drinks (coffee, soda, black tea, and green tea) in in different age groups (high school student, college student, adult, and elderly).

Regression analysis

Regression coefficient

- Regression coefficients represent the mean change in the outcome variable for one unit of change in the independent variable while holding other predictors constant.
- This statistical control that regression provides is important because it isolates the role of one variable from all of the others.
- It assumes a linear relationship between the variables.
- It cannot quantify the strength of the association between the two variables.

Linear regression analysis

- A linear regression analysis attempts to model the relationship between two variables (dependent variable by one or more independent variables) by fitting a linear equation to the observed data.
- *(Example: Depending on the variable: weight, Independent variable: height, BMI, and age)*
- A simplified straight line is drawn through the point cloud of the measurements (Fig. 11.2).

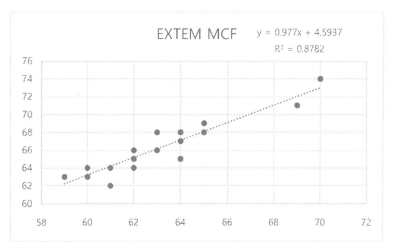

FIGURE 11.2 Extrinsic coagulation system (EXTEM) and maximum clot formation (MCF) via rotational thromboelastometry (ROTEM) analysis.

Example

Logistic regression

- The logistic regression is used for the analysis of dichotomous variables.

Example

Dependent variable: Heart attack [yes/no]
   Independent variable: Coffee [yes/no]
   Smoking [yes/no]

Poisson regression

- Poisson regression is used to model dependent variables that are counts. It tells you which explanatory variables have a statistically significant effect on the response variable.

- The concept of Poisson regression is based on the principle of linear regression.
- Poisson regression assumes the dependent variable has a Poisson distribution.
- The dependent variable are counts $(0, 1 \ldots \ldots n)$
- Number of new cases, number of deaths, number of attacks, number of polyps.

Example

Depending on the variable: number of polyps
   Independent variable: year

Survival analysis

- A survival analytical study consists of two periods:
  - Recruitment time
  - Follow-up time
- Patients admitted at the start of the recruitment period they have a maximum total observation time.
- Patients admitted at the end of the recruitment period they only have a minimum total observation time.

Censoring

- Censoring is common in survival analysis.
- Censoring is a form of missing data problem, in which the time to event is not observed for reasons such as termination of study before all recruited subjects have shown the event of interest, or the subject has left the study prior to experiencing an event.
- The survival time of an individual is censored when the endpoint is not observed during the study.
- If the exact time of death (end point) is known, it is considered for censoring.

Right censoring

- Loss to follow up, drop-out, end of study, death from another cause.

Left censoring

- The event occurred between the start of the study and the first examination date.

Interval censoring

- It is only known that the event occurred in interval A and B.

Kaplan Meier curve

- The Kaplan Meier curve is used to estimate the survival function that considers the dead or drop out (censored).

- The visual representation shows what the probability of survival is at a certain time interval.
- The Kaplan Meier curve lists survival according to the time and is not a statistical calculation.

Log-rank test
- The log-rank test is a comparison of two survival curves.
- Because the log-rank test is purely a test of significance it cannot provide an estimate of the size of the difference between the groups or a confidence interval.
- The P-value only gives information if the statistical difference between the groups is significant or not.
- The log-rank test is frequently used to determine the effect of a new therapy or drug to a control group.

Cox regression (proportional hazards regression)
- A log-rank test only gives only information if the difference between the groups is significant or not.
- A cox regression also calculates the relationship of effect between the groups.
- It is used for investigating the association between the survival time of patients and one or more independent variables.
- In a Cox proportional hazards regression model, the measure of effect is the hazard rate.
- The Hazard rate is the risk of failure (i.e., the risk or probability of suffering the event of interest).
- Hazard ratio (comparative measure), P-value
- Hazard ratio: A patient with a tumor stage T4 has, a XX times Hazard to die from the tumor.
- A hazard ratio above 1 indicates a covariate that is positively associated with the event probability, and thus negatively associated with the length of survival.
- $HR = 1$: No effect
- $HR < 1$: Reduction in the hazard
- $HR > 1$: Increase in Hazard

Correlation coefficient

- The correlation coefficient is a measure of the strength of the linear relationship between two variables (Figs. 11.3–11.7).

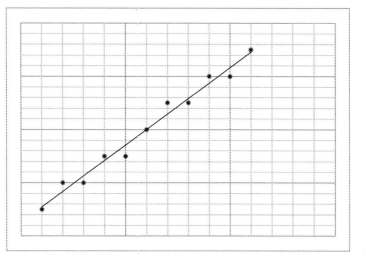

FIGURE 11.3   Positive strong correlation (close to correlation coefficient 1).

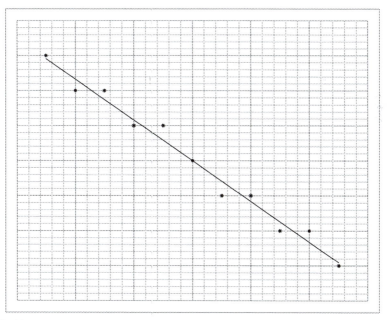

FIGURE 11.4   Negative strong correlation (close to correlation coefficient −1).

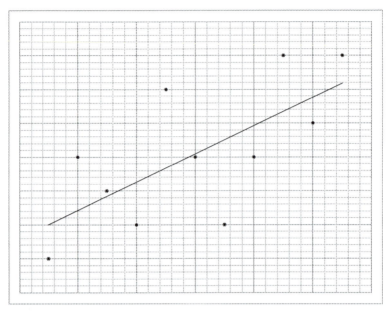

FIGURE 11.5 Positive weak correlation (correlation coefficient <1).

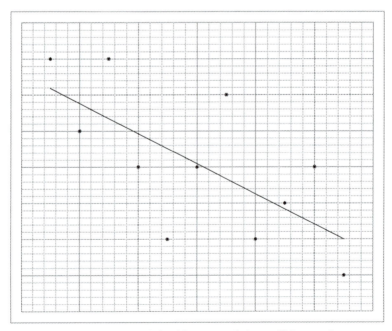

FIGURE 11.6 Negative weak correlation (close to correlation coefficient >−1).

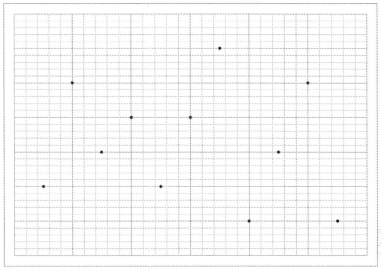

FIGURE 11.7   No correlation (correlation coefficient = 0).

- A correlation can be calculated when exposure and outcome are both being measured on a continuous scale.
- There are several types of correlation coefficient. Pearson's correlation (also called Pearson's R) is a correlation coefficient commonly used in linear regression.

Consistency measurements

Cronbach's alpha
- Cronbach's alpha is a measure of internal consistency, or the homogeneity of an assessment instrument (Table 11.3).

TABLE 11.3 Cronbach's alpha.

α	Interpretation of the alpha values
>0.9	Excellent
>0.8	Good
>0.7	Acceptable
>0.6	Questionable
>0.5	Bad
0.5	Unacceptable

- In other words, the reliability of any given measurement refers to the extent to which it is a consistent measure of a concept, and Cronbach's alpha is one way of measuring the strength of that consistency.
- It is often used for a test development or test evaluation.
- Cronbach's alpha is not a statistical test. It is a coefficient of reliability (or consistency).

Cohen's Kappa
- Cohen's kappa coefficient (κ) is a statistic that is used to measure inter-rater reliability (interobserver agreement) (Table 11.4).

TABLE 11.4 Cohen's kappa coefficient.

κ	Interpretation
<0	No agreement
0.0−0.20	Slight agreement
0.21−0.40	Fair agreement
0.41−0.60	Moderate agreement
0.61−0.80	Substantial agreement
0.81−1.00	Almost perfect agreement

- Hence the agreement between two raters (wo raters each rate one trial on each sample).
- Often used for systematic reviews.

Statistical errors

Regression to the mean

- Regression to the mean is the phenomenon that arises if a random variable is extreme on its first measurement but closer to the mean on its second measurement or observation.
- This effect occurs because a random unknown factor can influence the measurement or observation.
- This effect occurs more frequently if the variable is asymmetrically sampled from the population.
- The more extreme the sample group, the greater the regression to the mean.

Example

Patient A is participating in a blood pressure study. The mean of 100 subjects is 140/90.

In the first measurement, patient A has a blood pressure of 180/110.

The second measurement the next day measures a blood pressure of 150/90 and is therefore closer to the mean value of the study.

Multiple testing
- Multiple testing refers to the simultaneous testing of more than one hypothesis.
- The more outcomes or hypotheses are tested, the chance of getting a random significant result (statistical error) is high.
- If multiple testing is performed, there is typically a large probability that some of the true null hypotheses will be rejected.
- If statistical analysis is performed on all variables of the study there is a high change that a random statistical significant variable will be found.

Avoid multiple testing by
- The primary and secondary outcome should be clearly defined and not changed during the study.
- The primary outcome should be tested first.
- The secondary outcome should not be interpreted as an effect.

Example

Hypertension drug A is evaluated for the side effect.

Hypothesis: Drug A causes skin rash in contrast to placebo.

Primary outcome: rash

Secondary outcomes: rapid heartbeat, cough, headache, sweating, drowsiness, leg edema, abdominal pain, back pain....

The more secondary outcome measures are tested, the more likely to get a random significant result (multiple testing).

Statistical data presentation

- Statistically analyzed data should be presented in an effective format.
- The use of table and figures are an effective tool for comparison. It can reveal trends and relationships within the data such as changes over time, frequency distribution, and correlation.
- Statistical data should be presented in the result section of the manuscript.
- Primary outcome data should be presented first followed by the secondary outcome data.

Generally

- Round numbers and values.
- Depending on the statistics two or three digits after the decimal point is sufficient.
- Display the total number (N) together with the percentage.
- Display standard deviation with the mean values.

Frequency of distribution
- Patient characteristics.
- Age distribution (mean ± standard deviation)
- Gender distribution (percentage, number)
- BMI (mean ± standard deviation)

Significant values
- (P-value, lower CI—upper CI)
- (RR/OR, lower CI—upper CI)

Example

Overall, 200 patients were analyzed. The total we included 110 (55%) male and 90 (45%) females with a mean age of 51 ± 23 years. Among the 200 patients 174 pathological (2.32 ± 4.12 µg/L) and 26 nonpathological (0.069 ± 0.03 µg/L) serum S100B levels were reported. In 16 patients with traumatic brain injury the median levels of S100B were 0.581 ± 0.785 µg/L ($r = -0.107$, CI 0.824 to 2.232, $P < .001$).

Figures and table
- Figures and table are used to illustrate or present the main data more clearly to the reader.
- A figure should be simple, clear, and easy to understand.
- 2−3 figures in a manuscript are appropriate.
- 2−3 tables in a manuscript are appropriate.
- Most journals limit the amount of figures and tables in a publication.

Chapter 12

Random and systematic errors

Chapter outline

Random and systematic errors (Fig. 12.1)

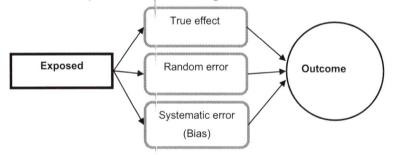

FIGURE 12.1 Cause of association between exposure and outcome effect.

Random error
- Random error describes the deviation of the results from the true value due to the unpredictability or uncertainty.

Causes
- There was a large variability in the measurement or population.
- These changes may occur in the measuring instruments or in the environmental conditions that are not controllable.

Systematic errors (bias)
- A systematic error is an error in design or implementation of the study that systematically causes the results to deviate from the true value.
- A systematic error is consistent and repeatable.

Causes
- The selection of subjects was different between the comparing groups.
- The study investigator had influences of the results.
- The study results were influenced by external factors (e.g., funding)

The Practical Guide to Clinical Research and Publication.
DOI: https://doi.org/10.1016/B978-0-12-824517-0.00007-1

Random versus systematic errors (Table 12.1; Figs. 12.2 and 12.3)

TABLE 12.1 Random error versus systematic error.

Random error	Systematic error
Results are not precise	Results are not valid (inaccurate)
Random error decreases/disappears with increase in sample size	Systematic error does not disappear with increase in sample size

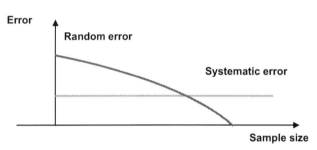

FIGURE 12.2 Systematic and random errors based on sample size.

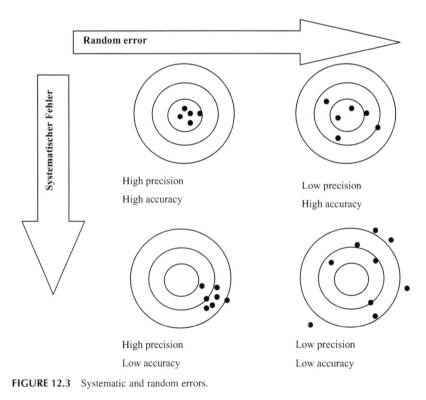

FIGURE 12.3 Systematic and random errors.

Bias

- Bias can lead to an association that is incorrect.
- A bias lead to either an overestimation or an underestimation of the true effect.
- Observational studies are particularly prone to bias.
- For example, those who are related to the disease are more interested in participating in the study than those who are not related to the disease.

Attrition bias

- Attrition bias is a systematic error or difference due to dropouts.
- It is caused unequal loss of participants (loss to follow up, drop out) in the groups (Fig. 12.4).

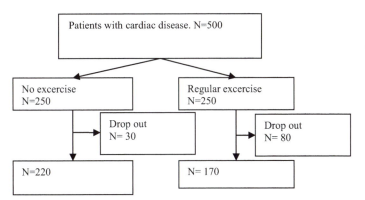

FIGURE 12.4   Attrition bias.

Performance bias

- A performance bias is a systematic difference in the treatment of the groups (apart from the intervention).
- Certain patients receive better medical care as part of a study, are monitored more closely or are given additional support (Fig. 12.5).

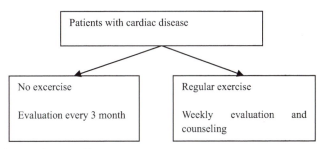

FIGURE 12.5   Performance bias.

Retrieval bias

- A retrieval bias is the incomplete finding of the publications in a systematic review.

Reporting bias

- A reporting bias is the difference in reported information about exposure/behavior /illness in each study groups.
- Cases (with severe or long-term illness) are better documented: more information on exposure is available.
- Participants hide undesirable/unaccepted behavior (drugs, alcohol consumption).
- Certain patient groups tend to under-document exposure (behavior analysis in obesity patients, smoking in pregnant women).

Recall bias

- A recall bias is when a study participant with a specific illness can remember more often about the event/risk exposure compared to a participant without a disease.
- This leads to differences in the accuracy or completeness of the recollections retrieved.
- A recall bias also leads to more frequent positive documentation in study participants with illness.
- Recall bias is a major problem in studies that have self-reporting, such as retrospective cohort studies.
- Case-control studies with self-reporting are especially vulnerable.

Detection bias

- It is the systematic difference in the outcome that results from closer observation of one group.
- Participants in a study group are examined more in detail compared to the control group.
- Therefore, more outcomes are discovered in the exposed group (more diseases are diagnosed).
- A detection bias can occur if the study investigator is not blinded.

Funding bias

- The results of a study are influenced by the funding organization (e.g., pharmaceutical company).

Language bias

- In systematic reviews or meta-analyzes, often only English studies are screened and selected.

- The results of systematic reviews and meta-analyzes are thereby distorted.

Publication bias
- Studies that can prove a positive effect are published more frequently.
- The entirety of the evidence is thereby biased and does not reflect the reality.

Research bias
- Is the possible bias in the evidence base due to the lack of valid studies.
- Mostly due to a lack of market interest.

Selection bias
- A selection bias is the systematic difference between the groups that are compared.
- Arises from the wrong group selection, different drop outs, etc. (Fig. 12.6).

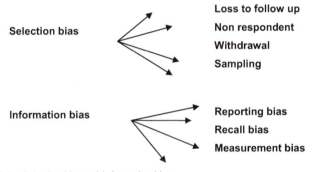

FIGURE 12.6   Selection bias and information bias.

Pygmalion effect
- Occurs when belief is influenced by an examiner's effect on study results.

Hawthorne effect
- Occurs when the test subjects know that they are taking part in the study and can influence the effect.

Confounders

- Confounding describes an association that is true but misleading (Fig. 12.7).

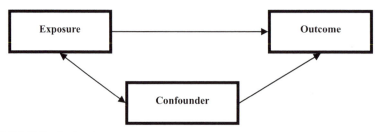

FIGURE 12.7 Confounder.

- Two conditions must be met for a confounder:
  - Relation to exposure without being a consequence of exposure
  - Relation to outcome regardless of exposure

  Confounder can be controlled by

- Randomizing, matching, stratification, specific selection of participants, stratified analysis, multivariable analysis (adjust).

Example (Fig. 12.8)

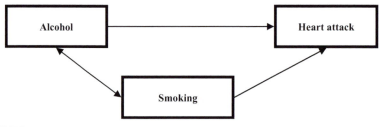

FIGURE 12.8 Example of confounder.

Example

One study examined alcohol consumption and heart attack (hypotheses: alcohol reduces the risk of heart attack).

Result: The group that consumes more alcohol has an increased risk of heart attack.

Reason: People with increased alcohol consumption are also smoking more frequently.

- *Alcohol does not increase the risk of heart attack.*
- *Smoking increases the risk of heart attack.*
- *Alcohol consumption and smoking are associated.*

  → this association masks the true context (Fig. 12.9)

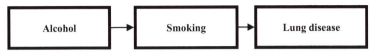

FIGURE 12.9 Not a confounder.

Example

Whole population (smoking and stroke)

Total	Cases	Controls	Total
Smokers	50	150	200
Nonsmokers	65	180	245
Total	115	330	445

$$OR = \frac{a/c}{b/d} = \frac{a^*d}{c^*b} = \frac{50^*180}{65^*150} = 0.92$$

Divided by gender: men

Men	Cases	Controls	Total
Smokers	28	131	159
Non-smokers	5	40	41
Total	33	171	200

$$OR = \frac{a/c}{b/d} = \frac{a^*d}{c^*b} = \frac{28^*40}{5^*131} = 1.71$$

Divided by gender: women

Women	Cases	Controls	Total
Smokers	22	29	50
Non-smokers	60	140	200
Total	82	169	250

$$OR = \frac{a/c}{b/d} = \frac{a^*d}{c^*b} = \frac{22^*140}{60^*29} = 1.77$$

- *OR* $_{Total} = 0,9$ *OR* $_{men} = 1.7$ *OR* $_{women} = 1.7$

  Gender is a confounder

- *Higher prevalence of the disease (stroke) in women.*
- *Most nonsmokers are women.*

Effect modification/interaction

- Effect modification occurs when the effects of exposure differ in the sub-groups (strata).

- OR (or RR) are different in the strata.
- Effect modification is not a bias, but important additional information.

Example: blood pressure and heart attack

O R_{total} = 1.5
O R_{men} = 1
O R_{women} = 2.5

Total, O R = 1.5

Total	Cases	Controls	Total
Blood pressure > 140	80	190	270
Blood pressure < 14 0	130	450	580
Total	210	640	850

Divided by age > 60, <60
Age < 60, O R = 1

Age > 60	Cases	Controls	Total
Blood pressure > 140	45	120	165
Blood pressure < 14 0	90	250	340
Total	135	370	505

Age > 60, O R = 2.5

Age <60	Cases	Controls	Total
Blood pressure > 140	35	70	105
Blood pressure < 140	40	200	240
Total	75	270	345

Age is an "effect modifier"

- *The magnitude of the effect of increased blood pressure on the risk of heart attack depends on age.*
- *An age > 60 is a major risk factor for heart attack in patients with blood pressure over 140.*

What to do with effect modification
- Stratification

Simpson's paradox
- The results of the subgroups can be different from the overall group:
  - Separate evaluation in subgroups.
  - Stratify (create strata-separated tables).
  - Calculate Mantel-Haenszel OR "(OR_{MH})/Mantel-Haenszel RR" (RR_{MH}).

Mantel-Haenszel odds ratio/relative risk

- Is a "combined" odds ratio/relative risk with a weighted average of the odds ratios of the individual categories.
- The weights are dependent on their size.

Stratification

- The aim is to form comparison groups that are homogeneous in themselves.
- In the stratification process, the population is divided into characteristics (gender, age, occupation, educational level, etc.), which should be considered in the participant enrollment phase.
- Stratification is problematic if there are too many variables (too many strata).
- Stratification is well suited for categorical variables.
- For continuous variables, a categorization is possible, but "residual confounding" may be present.
- Possibly a lower number of cases necessary.

Summary

Bias and confounding are a big problem in **observational studies**.
Difference between bias and confounder
- Bias leads to association that is wrong.
- Confounding describes an association that is true but misleading.
Confounders: OR, RR → equal in subgroup
Effect modification: OR, RR → different in subgroup

Chapter 13

Writing a manuscript and publication (Fig. 13.1)

Chapter outline

Purpose of scientific publishing

Scientific publishing

- The purpose of scientific publishing is to present the research result and to make it accessible to other scientists
- Freely accessible and exchange in information can lead to progress in science.
- However, publications and research information are often not freely accessible.
- Physicians and health-care scientists often have limited access to publications and scientific data.

Measure of career advancement

- The number of publication or impact factor is a requirement and measurement for academic achievement and promotion.
- There is constant competition between hospitals, research teams, professors, doctors and students to archive more publication.
- Due to the high publishing pressure, studies are often carried out improperly with the purpose of increasing the number of publications instead of the quality.
- People with limited scientific and research knowledge may conduct studies for career advancement.

The Practical Guide to Clinical Research and Publication.
DOI: https://doi.org/10.1016/B978-0-12-824517-0.00009-5

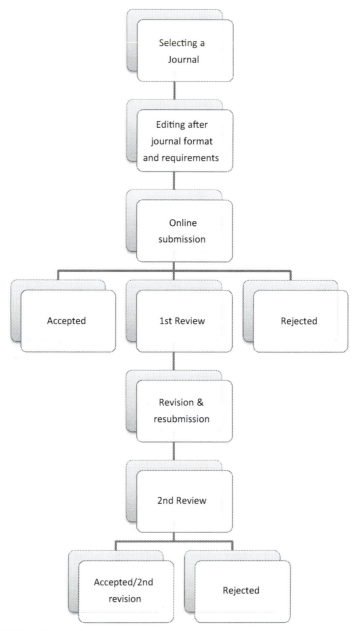

FIGURE 13.1 Publication process.

Influence of the publishing industry on publications

- The publishing industry, like all other business, is subject to capitalism and the market economy, and supply and demand principle.

- Research for publication is selected based on the current research trend.
- Studies with low audience interest are less considered for publication.
- For marketing purposes every month new journals are created or renamed. Not all new journals survive.
- Researchers and publishing companies are funded for publication if there is a specific interest in a research topic.

Influence of the pharmaceutical companies on publications
- A study result may be published in favor of the funder.
- Studies that may harm the product or the company are not published.
- Studies are used for advertising and marketing purposes.
- Only studies that are in the company's own interest will be funded.

Largest medicine publisher
Elsevier
- Is a division of Reed Elsevier PLC and is the largest company in the medical journaling industry.
- Reed Elsevier PLC revenue was 7874 billion GBP(10.69 billion USD) in 2019
- Elsevier owns over 2500 journals and about 20,000 books
  - EMBASE Online Database (7600 biomedical journals from 90 countries)
  - ScienceDirect Online Datenbank
  - MD Consult
  - Lancet
  - And many more

Example

The following journals are listed under the category Surgery (Elsevier publishing)

Aesthetic Surgery Journal
Annals of Vascular Surgery
Asian Journal of Surgery
British Journal of Oral and Maxillofacial Surgery
Clinics in Plastic Surgery
European Journal of Cardio-Thoracic Surgery
European Journal of Vascular and Endovascular Surgery
European Urology
International Journal of Oral and Maxillofacial Surgery
Journal of Cranio-Maxillofacial Surgery
Journal of Oral and Maxillofacial Surgery
Journal of Pediatric Surgery
Journal of Plastic, Reconstructive & Aesthetic Surgery
Journal of Vascular Surgery

Journal of the American College of Surgeons
Surgery
The Journal of Heart and Lung Transplantation
The American Journal of Surgery
And many more...

Finding the appropriate journal

Journal
- There are hundreds of journals for a single subject or research topic.
- It is important to find the appropriate journal to submit your research to reach the right audience.
- The research topic should match the scope of the journal and audience.
- A major reason for the rejection is that the research topic does not fit with the journal scope.

Screening
- Which journals is the best fit for my research topic? (Table 13.1)
  - Search for journals in the library
  - Search online for journal lists for the research topic
  - Search for a journal where a similar study has been published before
  - Seek consultation from colleagues who have experience in that topic
  - Discuss with specialists in the area

Impact factor

- The impact factor (IF) is a measure of the frequency with which the average article in a journal has been cited in a particular year. It is used to measure the importance or rank of a journal by calculating the times it's articles are cited.
- The calculation is based on a two-year period. It divides the number of cited articles by the number of published articles.

$$\text{Impact Factor} = \frac{\text{Number of citation in the last two years}}{\text{Number of published articles in the last two years}}$$

Example

A journal published a total of 100 articles in the years 2019–2020.
In 2008 articles were 300 cited 300 times.

$$\text{Impact Factor} = \frac{300}{100} = 3$$

The journals impact factor for 2019 is 3.00

TABLE 13.1 Checklist for journal screening.

Criteria	Yes/no
Does the impact factor and "Journal prestige" meet the expectations of the author?	
Is the Journal PubMed listed?	
Open access journal versus nonopen accessed journal. Is it an established journal?	
Does my university/institution have access to the journal?	
Is the research that will be submitted a laboratory or clinical research?	
Is the topic of the research to be submitted similar to the Journal focus?	
Is the review process supportive (adequate criticism, timely)?	
How fast is the publication process?	
Are there publication fees?	
Do you know the journal editor?	
Are you interested in supporting the organization that publishes the journal? What is the rejection rate.	

The journal can deliberately reduce the number of publications or influence the number of citations and thus increase the impact factor.

Journal rankings

Journal citation reports

- Journal citation reports provides ranking for journals in the areas of science, technology, and social sciences.
- For every journal covered, the following information is collected or calculated: citation and article counts, impact factor, immediacy index, cited half-life, citing half-life, source data listing, citing journal listing, cited journal listing, subject categories, publisher information.
- Limited to the citation data of Journals indexed in Web of Science.
- Process to determine journals included in the tool.
- Indexes over 12,000 journals in arts, humanities, sciences, and social sciences.

SCImago journal rank (SJR)

- The SCImago journal & Country Rank is a portal that includes the journals and country scientific indicators developed from the information contained in the Scopus® database (Elsevier B.V.).
- Scopus contains more than 15,000 journals from over 4000 international publishers as well as over 1000 open access journals.
- SCImago's "evaluation of scholarly journals is to assign weights to bibliographic citations based on the importance of the journals that issued them, so that citations issued by more important journals will be more valuable than those issued by less important ones" (SJR indicator).

Scopus (Elsevier)

- The Scopus Journal Analyzer provides a view of journal performance, enriched with two journal metrics—SJR (SCImago Journal Rank) and SNIP (Source Normalized Impact per Paper).
- Over 15,000 journals from over 4000 international publishers.

Journal of a specific medical specialty

Example

Various cardiology journals and their impact factor

Journal name	JCR data		
	Total citation	Impact factor	5 year impact factor
Circulation	151,045	**14.432**	14.932
Journal of the American College of Cardiology	69,411	**14.293**	13.091
European Heart Journal	26,318	**10.052**	10.085
Circulation Research	42,346	**9.504**	10.190
Nature Reviews Cardiology	440	**7.467**	7.467
International Journal of Cardiology	11,529	**6.802**	4.004
Journal of Heart Valve Disease	1866	**0.927**	1.178
Journal of Cardiothoracic Surgery	232	**0.908**	0.977
Scandinavian Cardiovascular Journal	539	**0.895**	1.048

Top impact factor journal (Table 13.2)

TABLE 13.2 Medical journals listed according to high impact factor.

	Journal title	JCR data			
		Total citation	Impact factor	5 year impact factor	Cited articles
1	CA-A Cancer Journal for Clinicians	9804	**94.333**	70.245	18
2	New England Journal of Medicine	227,679	**53.486**	52.363	345
3	Annual Review of Immunology	16,100	**49.271**	46.688	22
4	Nature Reviews Molecular Cell Biology	26,838	**38.650**	41.578	70
5	Nature Reviews Cancer	26,729	**37.184**	37.881	71
6	Nature Genetics	76,301	**36.377**	32.701	178
7	Nature	511,248	**36.104**	35.248	862
8	Nature Reviews Immunology	21,080	**35.196**	33.644	70
9	Lancet	155,736	**33.633**	32.498	271
10	Cell	167,591	**32.406**	34.931	319
11	Science	469,815	**31.377**	31.777	862
12	JAMA-Journal of the American Medical Association	117,497	**30.011**	29.310	233

April, 2012.

Scientific writing

Good research alone is not enough for publication. The research needs to be presented in a comprehensible way in scientific writing.

Authorship

Authorship
- Sequence: first author, coauthor / second author, coauthor 1, coauthor 2 . . ., senior author.
- Authorship confers credit and has important academic, social, and financial implications.

- The lead author is of particular importance for an academic career.
- Authorship also implies responsibility and accountability for published work.
- Always clarify the order of authorship with all coauthors before starting your research.
- To avoid disputes in some research groups no names but only the research group is listed.
- Because authorship does not communicate what contributions qualified an individual to be an author, some journals now request and publish information about the contributions of each person named as having participated in a submitted study, at least for original research.
- Editors are strongly encouraged to develop and implement a contributorship policy.
- Such policies remove much of the ambiguity surrounding contributions but leave unresolved the question of the quantity and quality of contribution that qualify an individual for authorship.
- The ICMJE (international committee of medical journal editors) has thus developed criteria for authorship that can be used by all journals, including those that distinguish authors from other contributors.

Who is an author?

The ICMJE (international committee of medical journal editors) recommends that authorship be based on the following four criteria:
1. Substantial contributions to the conception or design of the work; or the acquisition, analysis, or interpretation of data for the work; AND
2. Drafting the work or revising it critically for important intellectual content; AND
3. Final approval of the version to be published; AND
4. Agreement to be accountable for all aspects of the work in ensuring that questions related to the accuracy or integrity of any part of the work are appropriately investigated and resolved.

Nonauthor contributors

- Contributors who meet fewer than all four of the above criteria for authorship should not be listed as authors, but they should be acknowledged.
- Examples of activities that alone (without other contributions) do not qualify a contributor for authorship are acquisition of funding; general supervision of a research group or general administrative support; and writing assistance, technical editing, language editing, and proofreading.
- Those whose contributions do not justify authorship may be acknowledged individually or together as a group.

http://www.icmje.org/recommendations/browse/roles-and-responsibilities/defining-the-role-of-authors-and-contributors.html

Abstract

- An abstract is a short summary of the research to give the reader a complete and concise understanding of the research findings.
- The abstract should follow a clear structure, background, methods, results conclusion.
- An abstract should contain approximately 250—500 words.
- Different checklists and criteria are available to help writing a structured abstract (Table 13.3).

TABLE 13.3 CONSORT criteria for an abstract.

Item	Description
Title	Identification of the study as randomized
Authors	Contact details for the corresponding author
Trial design	Description of the trial design (e.g., Parallel, cluster, non-inferiority)
Methods	
Participants	Eligibility criteria for participants and the settings where the data were collected
Intervention	Interventions intended for each group
Objective	Specific objective or hypothesis
Outcome	Clearly defined primary outcome for this report
Randomization	How participants were allocated to interventions
Blinding (masking)	Whether or not participants, care givers, and those assessing the outcomes were blinded to group assignment
Results	
Numbers randomized	Number of participants randomized to each group
Recruitment	Trial status
Numbers analyzed	Number of participants analyzed in each group
Outcome	For the primary outcome, a result for each group and the estimated effect size and its precision
Harms	Important adverse events or side effects
Conclusions	General interpretation of the results
Trial registration	Registration number and name of the trial register
Funding	Source of funding

Importance of an abstract
- The importance of an abstract is often underestimated.
- In addition to the title, an abstract is the most read part of an article and the one that is most easily accessible to a reader.
- In many areas of the world, doctors and health care related scientists have restricted access to publications and often only to abstracts.
- For systematic reviews, meta-analyzes and HTA reports (Health Technology Assessment), which represent the highest level in the evidence hierarchy, the abstract is of enormous importance because the decision to include / exclude a study is made based on abstract screening.

Manuscript

- A manuscript should contain and summarize the most important information of the research.
- It usually follows the format of, introduction, methods, results discussion, and conclusion.
- Several checklists are available that can help writing a manuscript while focusing on the important aspects of each section (Table 13.4).

TABLE 13.4 Statements and checklists for reporting quality improvement in studies.

CONSORT	Randomized control trial
STROBE	Observational studies
PRISMA	Meta-analysis: randomized controlled trial, systematical review
STARD	Studies of diagnostic accuracy
MOOSE	Meta-analysis of observational studies in epidemiology
REMARK	(Reporting recommendations for tumor marker prognostic studies)
STARLITE	Standards for reporting literature searches
TREND	Transparent reporting of evaluations with nonrandomized designs

Manuscript format

Introduction
- Background information, hypothesis, and introduction.

Methods
- Study planning, patient selection, outcomes, and statistics.

- Use flowchart if necessary.

Result
- Presentation of the results. Primary outcome and secondary outcome.
- No comments or reviews.
- Use illustration and tables.
- Pay attention to the accuracy of the data.

Discussion
- Summarize the main results.
- Explanation of the results found.
- Strengths, weaknesses of the study
- Limitation (bias, confounder) of the study

Conclusion
- Assessment of results and research approach in the future
- Make short (2–5 sets)

Common mistakes in writing a manuscript
- Inadequate English, grammatical error, not formatted to journal requirement
- Sentences are too long and incomprehensible
- No flow between paragraphs
- Repeating the data in "Result"
- Incorrect interpretation of the results found
- Results not sufficiently discussed
- Irrelevant or incorrect discussion approach
- No description of the weaknesses/limitation of the study
- Conclusion does not support the results of the study
- Missing references

Reference

- A reference is the list of the cited articles in the manuscript.
- All references should be uniform and follow a specific format.
- Each journal has a preference of the reference format. Specific information can be found under "Author guidelines" in each journal.

Reference style
- AMA (American Medical Association)
- APA (American Psychological Association)
- Chicago
- Harvard
- IEEE (Institute for Electrical and Electronics Engineers)
- MLA (Modern Language Association)
- Vancouver

MEDLINE®/PubMed® Journal reference format
(ANSI/NISO Z39.29-2005 (R2010) Bibliographic References standard)
Name: followed by a comma.
Author initials: in capital letters, between the authors comma, followed by period.
Full title of the article: first letter in large, at the end period.
Full title of journal: in abbreviation, first letter in large, then period.
Year, month and date of publication: followed by semicolon.
Volume number
Issue/Part number: in brackets, followed by a colon.
Number of pages: then dot.
PMID: enter PubMed identification number.

Example

Yoon U, Topper J, Goldhammer J. Preoperative evaluation and anesthetic management of patients with liver cirrhosis undergoing cardiac surgery. J Cardiothorac Vasc Anesth 2020 Aug 14:S1053–0770(20)30816–8. doi: 10.1053/j.jvc.2020.08.022. Epub ahead of print. PMID: 32891522.

Internet references format
URL (last access date)

Example

http://de.wikipedia.org/wiki/medicine *(6.10.2021)*

Reference-managing computer programs
- Using a reference managing software can be helpful, especially in review articles.
- The cited literature can be directly imported from PubMed, websites or as PDF.
- All journal reference formats are presaved and an adjustment of all cited reference is easy.
- Reference Manager®, JabRef®, Mendeley.

Journal submission

- Once the manuscript if finalized and the appropriate journal selected it can be submitted.
- Currently most journals accept online submission only (Fig. 13.2).

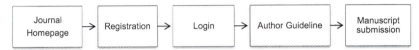

FIGURE 13.2   Manuscript submission.

ORCID ID

- ORCID is a nonprofit organization helping create a world in which all who participate in research, scholarship and innovation are uniquely identified and connected to their contributions and affiliations, across disciplines, borders, and time.
- ORCID provides a persistent digital identifier (an ORCID D) for the registered user.
- The ID can be connected with the user's professional information—affiliations, grants, publications, peer review, and more.
- The ID can be used to share the user's information with other systems and journal submission platforms.

Author guideline

- Each journal has specific requirements how to format a manuscript. The "Author guideline," usually found on the homepage, contains the most important information for the author.
- Manuscripts that are not following the journals specific formatting guideline is a major reason for rejection.
- The manuscript should be corrected and reviewed before each journal submission if it is consistent with the "Author guideline".
- Many journals also require the following documents upon submission:
  - Cover letter
  - Delaraton of authorship
  - Signed statements form everyone listed as author
  - Statement of conflict of interest
  - Patient consent form (case report)

Conflicts of interest

- The purpose of Conflicts of Interest is to provide readers of the manuscript with information about other interests that could influence how they receive and understand the work.
- Each author should submit a separate form and is responsible for the accuracy and completeness of the submitted information.

- Electronic conflict of interest form can be found at http://www.icmje.org/conflicts-of-interest/.

Review process

Peer review
- Reviewers play a pivotal role in scholarly publishing.
- The peer review system exists to validate academic work, helps to improve the quality of published research, and increases networking possibilities within research communities.
- Peer review is designed to assess the validity, quality and often the originality of articles for publication.
- Peer review has been a formal part of scientific communication since the first scientific journals appeared more than 300 years ago.
- Despite criticisms, peer review is still the only widely accepted method for research validation and has continued successfully with relatively minor changes.
- The Philosophical Transactions of the Royal Society is thought to be the first journal to formalize the peer review process under the editorship of Henry Oldenburg (1618–1677).
- Despite many criticisms about the integrity of peer review, the majority of the research community still believes peer review is the best form of scientific evaluation.

Single blind review
- In this type of review, the names of the reviewers are hidden from the author. This is the traditional method of reviewing and is the most common type by far.
- Points to consider regarding single blind review include:
  - Reviewer anonymity allows for impartial decisions—the reviewers should not be influenced by the authors.
  - Authors may be concerned that reviewers in their field could delay publication, giving the reviewers a chance to publish first.
  - Reviewers may use their anonymity as justification for being unnecessarily critical or harsh when commenting on the authors' work.

Double-blind review
- Both the reviewer and the author are anonymous in this model.
- Advantages of this model are listed below.
- Author anonymity limits reviewer bias, for example based on an author's gender, country of origin, academic status or previous publication history.
  - Articles written by prestigious or renowned authors are considered on the basis of the content of their papers, rather than their reputation.

- Despite the above, reviewers can often identify the author through their writing style, subject matter or self-citation. It is exceedingly difficult to guarantee total author anonymity.

Triple-blind review

- With triple-blind review, reviewers are anonymous and the author's identity is unknown to both the reviewers and the editor.
- Articles are anonymized at the submission stage and are handled in such a way to minimize any potential bias towards the authors.
- The complexities involved with anonymizing articles/authors to this level are considerable.
- as with double-blind review; there is still a possibility for the editor and/or reviewers to correctly recognize the author's identity from their style, subject matter, citation patterns or a number of other methodologies.

Open review

- Open peer review is an umbrella term for many different models aiming at greater transparency during and after the peer review process.
- The most common definition of open review is when both the reviewer and author are known to each other during the peer review process.
- Other types of open peer review consist of:
  - Publication of reviewers' names on the article page.
  - Publication of peer review reports alongside the article, whether signed or anonymous.
  - Publication of peer review reports (signed or anonymous) together with authors' and editors' responses alongside the article.
  - Publication of the paper after a quick check and opening a discussion forum to the community who can comment (named or anonymous).
  - Many believe this is the best way to prevent malicious comments, stop plagiarism, prevent reviewers from following their own agenda, and encourage open, honest reviewing. Others see open review as a less honest process, in which politeness or fear of retribution may cause a reviewer to withhold or tone down criticism.

Review process

- The submitted manuscript is sent to $2-3$ independent reviewers using the peer review process (Fig. 13.3).
- They independently comments on the manuscript with an overall recommendation (accept, reject, minor changes, major changes)
- If all reviewers are in agreement that the manuscript is not sufficient for publication, it will get rejected.
- If the reviewers' opinions are inconsistent, another reviewer is usually consulted or the editor in chief makes the final decision.

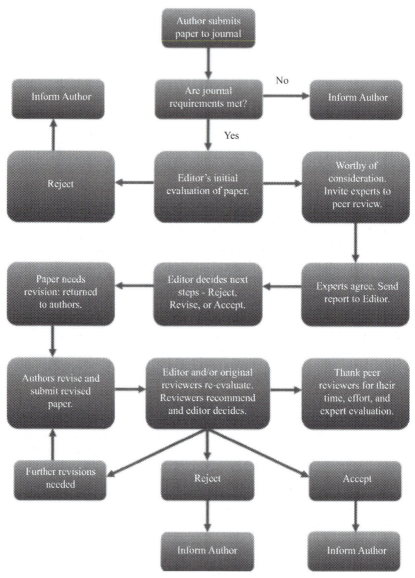

FIGURE 13.3   Jounal submission flowhcart.

Assessment criteria
1. Originality, methodology and presentation
2. Overall assessment (top 10%, top 25%, top 50%, bottom 50%, rejected)
3. Reviewer comment to the editor

4. Reviewer comment to the author
- Is the manuscript acceptable but not sufficient for the publication, a commentary list is created by each reviewer.
- Each individual point must be specifically answered and changed in the manuscript.

Peer review disadvantages
- The reviewer is mostly anonymous.
- Not every reviewer has the topic related specific knowledge and can make a clear judgement.
- Medical professionals are rarely trained in clinical epidemiology or biometrics.
- Epidemiologic or biometric professionals are rarely medically trained.
- Is peer review objective or subjective? (Table 13.5).

TABLE 13.5 Peer review focus of the reviewers depending on their qualifications.

Reviewer	Main focus
Medical professionals	Clinical focus, discussion
Native English reviewer	Grammar, spelling
Public health specialist	Public health relevant topic
Epidemiologist	Study design, methodology
Statistician	Statistics
Librarian	References

https://www.elsevier.com/reviewers/what-is-peer-review.

Revision
- Usually two revisions are permitted.
- If the author fails to make adequate revision during this time to improve the manuscript it may get rejected.

Example of a review process

Reviewer's report title: Manuscript 1
   Version: 1 **Date:** February 1, 2011 **Reviewer:** 1
   Reviewer's report:

(Continued)

(Continued)

Overall, this is an interesting paper that provides useful information about the quality of abstracts presented in a congress of burn medicine. The research builds on prior work reported by the authors in the literature, and this is a strength, as is much of the study design. Nevertheless, a number of concerns dampen enthusiasm for accepting the paper in its current version. These are listed below.

Major compulsory revisions

The number of abstracts analyzed is not clear since the authors mention 259 abstracts in 2000 and 252 in 2008, but they seems to have excluded 81 experimental studies in 2000 and 74 experimental studies in 2008. The percentages are calculated on the total number of abstracts and not on the abstracts analyzed.

This should be clarified.

Author response: We clarified this and add in the abstract and result: Overall 511 abstracts (2000: N = 259, 2008: N = 252) were screened. 13 RCT's in 2000 and 9 in 2008, 77 observational studies in 2000 and 98 in 2008 were included for scoring.

The authors should discuss other tools to assess the quality of abstracts presented in meeting, particularly the rate of subsequent publication in peer reviewed journals.

Author response: The problem-what that there what no other tool to assess the reporting quality in abstracts. We discussed this in the limitation part. We didn't mention about the full-text publication rate because this was not the issue in this study.

Minor essential revisions

References In some of them the month is mentioned, but not in all. The journal is sometimes underlines. The last page is sometimes in full, sometimes not. Harmonization is needed.

Discretionary revisions none

Author's response: We reviewed the references.

Level of interest: An article of limited interest

Quality of written English: Needs some language corrections before being published

Statistical review: Yes, and I have assessed the statistics in my report.

Declaration of competing interests: I declare that I have no competing interests

Journal rejection

Acceptance rate

- Highly regarded general journals 1%−20%
- Subject-specific journals 10%−30%
- Other specialist journals 30%−50%

- New journals 40%−70%
- Paid journals 70%−90%

Reasons for rejection

- More studies are submitted for publication than the journal can publish.
- A journal has preferences. For example, for laboratory research or clinical research.
- The research question, topic or methodology does not fit the journal focus.
- Statistics is questionable in order to be interpreted as valid.
- Inadequate English and grammatical errors.
- Review process between reviewer and author cannot improve the manuscript to be adequate for publication.

Declined

- If a study is rejected, a journal with a lower impact factor is usually searched for to resubmission.
- Re-formatting according to the journal format can be time-consuming and tedious for the clinician.
- Time is a big factor for clinicians and researchers and they may choose not to further try resubmission.

Further literature

- Albert T. Winning the publications game. 2nd ed. Radcliffe Medical Publishing; July 2000. ISBN-10: 1857754719.
- Albert T. How to handle authorship disputes: a guide for new researchers http://publicationethics.org/files/u2/2003pdf12.pdf.
- http://www.nature.com/nature/peerreview/debate/index.html.
- Parmley WW. Why did JACC reject my manuscript? J Am Coll Cardiol 2001;37(1):323−4.

Chapter 14

Critical literature review

Chapter outline

Not everything is evidence

> ... Some (the purists would say 99%) of published articles belong in the bin...
> *Greenhalgh (2001)*

Critical literature review
- The critical literature review is an essential component of evidence-based medicine (Fig. 14.1).
- It provides a systematic evaluation of research weighting up the advantages and disadvantages, strengths, and weaknesses.
- The quality of a literature can be assessed with checklists.
- A critical literature review can identify poor studies that may falsify the evidence.
- A critical literature review is important to avoid making clinical decisions based on poorly conducted studies.
- 45.

Includes
- Analyze reporting quality of manuscripts.
- Distinguish methodologically well conducted from poorly conducted studies.
- Recognize lacking knowledge in study design.
- Detect and analyze misinterpretation.
- Recognize the influence of funding.
- Analyze the applicability of the studies in evidence-based medicine.

The Practical Guide to Clinical Research and Publication.
DOI: https://doi.org/10.1016/B978-0-12-824517-0.00001-0

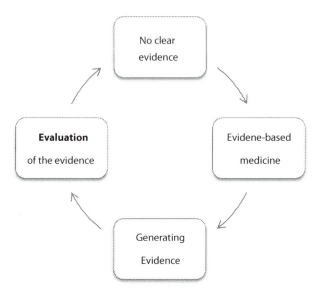

FIGURE 14.1 Critical literature review.

High quality clinical trial
- Quality = level of evidence (study design) + research quality

  A high-quality study should have:

- A clear research question.
- Study design and implementation in accordance with epidemiological and biometric standards.
- A high internal validity.
- A high external validity.
- Clear data analysis and transparent presentation.

Report quality & methodical quality

Reporting quality
- In order to assess the reporting quality, the completeness of information is checked without assessing the information for validity.
- It is important that the research is reported in a transparent manner. The reader should be able to understand how the research was planned, conducted and what the primary outcome and conclusion is.

- It is possible that poorly described studies have been carried out with good methodological quality and conversely that well-described studies have poor methodological qualities.
- If information is missing, it cannot be differentiated whether it was not considered in the study design or was just not reported in the publication.
- A lack of language skills can affect the reporting quality.

Methodological quality

- Methodological quality refers to an effort in a study to minimize bias.
- In order to evaluate the methodological quality, features of the design, implementation and statistical analysis of a research study can be used.
- However, the methodological quality of a study can only be properly evaluated if it has been clearly and transparently described (good reporting quality).
- A good reporting quality is therefore a prerequisite for the analysis of the methodological quality.
- The credibility of a study depends on third parties being able to critically assess the strengths and weaknesses of the study design, implementation, and evaluation.

Abstract

Reporting quality
- Measuring instrument: CONSORT for Abstract, Timmer Score (validated)

Methodological quality
- It is difficult to assess the methodological quality of a study based on the abstract, since an abstract is mostly limited to <500 words and therefore only contains the most important information.
- Measuring instrument: Timmer Score (validated)

Manuscript

Report quality
- Measuring instruments (Table 14.1):

TABLE 14.1 Statements and checklists for reporting quality improvement in studies.

CONSORT	Randomised controlled trial
STROBE	Observational studies
PRISMA	Meta-analyse: randomized controlled trial, systematical review
STARD	Studies of diagnostic accuracy
MOOSE	Meta-analysis of observational studies in epidemiology
REMARK	(REporting recommendations for tumor MARKer prognostic studies)
STARLITE	(Standards for Reporting Literature searches)
TREND	Transparent reporting of evaluations with nonrandomized designs

Methodological quality
- Measuring instruments (Table 14.2):

TABLE 14.2 Methodological quality measuring instruments.

Instrument	Application
Sign 50	Methodology checklist 1: systematic reviews and meta-analysis Methodology checklist 2: randomized controlled trials Methodology checklist 3: Cohort studies Methodology checklist 4: Case-control studies Methodology checklist 5: Diagnostic studies
NHS CASP (Critical appraisal skills program)	12 questions to help you make sense of a diagnostic test study 11 questions to help you make sense of a case control study 12 questions to help you make sense of a cohort study 10 questions to help you make sense of randomized controlled trials 10 questions to help you make sense of reviews
Jadad scale (Oxford scale)	Randomized controlled trials
IQWIG	Quality assessment: diagnostic studies

Further reading

- CONSORT-statement: http://www.consort-statement.org
- CONSORT for abstract: Hopewell S, et al. Better reporting of randomized trials in biomedical journal and conference abstracts. J Inf Sci 2008;34:162−73. STROBE-Statement: von Elm E, Altman DG, Egger M, Pocock SJ, Gotzsche PC, Vandonbroucke JP für die STROBE-initiative. Das strengthening the reporting of observational studies in epidemiology (STROBE-)statement. Leitlinien für das Berichten von Beobachtungsstudien. Internist 2008;49:688−93.
- QUOROM-statement: improving the quality of reports of meta-analyses of randomised controlled trials: the QUOROM statement (Moher et al. The Lancet 1999).
- PRISMA-statement: Moher D, Liberati A, Tetzlaff J, Altman DG; PRISMA Group. Preferred reporting items for systematic reviews and meta-analyses: the PRISMA statement. BMJ 2009;339:b2535.
- MOOSE-statement: Meta-analyse of observational studies in epidemiology: a proposal for reporting (Stromp et al. JAMA 2000).
- STARD-statement: towards complete and accurate reporting of studies of diagnostic accuracy: the STARD initiative (Bossuyt et al. Clinical Chemistry 2003).
- REMARK-statement: McShane LM, Altman DG, Sauerbrei W, et al. Reporting recommendations for tumor MARKer prognostic studies (REMARK). Nat Clin Pract Oncol 2005;2(8):416−22.
- STARLITE-statement: Booth A "Brimful of STARLITE": toward standards for reporting literature searches. J Med Libr Assoc 2006 Oct;94(4):421−9, e205. PMID: 17082834 (PubMed − indexed for MEDLINE).
- TREND-statement: Des Jarlais DC, Lyles C, Crepaz N, and the TREND Group. Improving the reporting quality of nonrandomized evaluations of behavioral and public health interventions: the TREND statement. Am J Public Health 2004;94:361−6.
- JADAD-score: Jadad AR et al. Assessing the quality of reports of randomized clinical trials: is blinding necessary? Control Clin Trials 1996;17(1):1−12. Timmer A, Sutherland LR, Hilsden RJ. Development and evaluation of a quality score for abstracts. BMC Med Res Methodol 2003;3:2. Epub February 11, 2003.

Chapter 15

Checklist for quality assessment

Chapter outline

Timmer score (Table 15.1)

TABLE 15.1 Timmer score.

Quality assessment		yes	partial	no	n/a
1.	Question / objective sufficiently described?				
2.	Design evident and appropriate to answer study question?				
3.	Subject characteristics sufficiently described?				
4.	Subjects appropriate to the study question?				
5.	Controls used and appropriate? **(if no control, check no)**				
6.	Method of subject selection described and appropriate?				
7.	If random allocation to treatment groups was possible, is it described? (if not possible, check n/a)				
8.	If blinding of investigators to intervention was possible, is it reported? (If not possible, n/a)				
9.	If blinding of subjects to intervention was possible, is it reported? (If not possible, n/a)[1]				
10.	Outcome measure well defined and robust to measurement bias? Means of assessment reported?				
11.	Confounding accounted for?				
12.	Sample size adequate?				
13.	Post hoc power calculations or confidence intervals reported for statistically non significant results?				
14.	Statistical analyses appropriate?				
15.	Statistical tests stated?				
16.	Exact p-values or confidence intervals stated?				
17.	Attrition of subjects and reason for attrition recorded?				
18.	Results reported in sufficient detail?				
19.	Do the results support the conclusions?				
Sum (items 1-19)					

Scoring: For each applicable item, 0−1 points are awarded (1 if met, 0 if not met). For each item which is not applicable, such as blinding of subjects in observational trials, items are subtracted from the total possible score. The summary score is calculated by summate the score of each item.

The Practical Guide to Clinical Research and Publication.
DOI: https://doi.org/10.1016/B978-0-12-824517-0.00006-X

Jadad scale

- Methodological quality assessment for randomized controlled studies
- A maximum of 5 points can be achieved (Table 15.2)

TABLE 15.2 Jadad scale.

	Points	description
Randomization	1	Was the study described as randomized?
	+ 1	Was the method of randomization appropriate?
	-1	Was the method randomization inappropriate?
Blinding	1	The study was described as double-blind
	+ 1	Was the method of blinding appropriate?
	- 1	Was the method of blinding inappropriate?
drop-out	1	Was there a description of withdrawals and dropouts?

Benefits
- Easy to use
- Validated instrument

Disadvantage
- Mainly focuses only on randomization, blinding, and drop-outs
- Limited assessability of a study

Consort for abstract—items to include when reporting a randomized trial in a journal or conference abstract (Table 15.3)

TABLE 15.3 Consort for abstracts.

Item	Description	Reported (yes/no)
Title	Identification of the study as randomized	
Authors *	Contact details for the corresponding author	
Trial design	Description of the trial design (e.g. parallel, cluster, non-inferiority)	
Methods		
Participants	Eligibility criteria for participants and the settings where the data were collected	
Interventions	Interventions intended for each group	
Objective	Specific objective or hypothesis	
Outcome	Clearly defined primary outcome for this report	
Randomization	How participants were allocated to interventions	
Blinding (masking)	Whether or not participants, care givers, and those assessing the outcomes were blinded to group assignment	
Results		
Numbers randomized	Number of participants randomized to each group	
Recruitment	Trial status	
Numbers analysed	Number of participants analysed in each group	
Outcome	For the primary outcome, a result for each group and the estimated effect size and its precision	
Harms	Important adverse events or side effects	
Conclusions	General interpretation of the results	
Trial registration	Registration number and name of trial register	
Funding	**Source of funding**	

*This item is specific to conference abstracts.

CONSORT statement (Table 15.4)

TABLE 15.4 Checklist for randomized controlled trials.

Section/Topic	Item No	Checklist item
Title and abstract		
	1a	Identification as a randomised trial in the title
	1b	Structured summary of trial design, methods, results, and conclusions (for specific guidance see CONSORT for abstracts)
Introduction		
Background and objectives	2a	Scientific background and explanation of rationale
	2b	Specific objectives or hypotheses
Methods		
Trial design	3a	Description of trial design (such as parallel, factorial) including allocation ratio
	3b	Important changes to methods after trial commencement (such as eligibility criteria), with reasons
Participants	4a	Eligibility criteria for participants
	4b	Settings and locations where the data were collected
Interventions	5	The interventions for each group with sufficient details to allow replication, including how and when they were actually administered
Outcomes	6a	Completely defined pre-specified primary and secondary outcome measures, including how and when they were assessed
	6b	Any changes to trial outcomes after the trial commenced, with reasons
Sample size	7a	How sample size was determined
	7b	When applicable, explanation of any interim analyses and stopping guidelines
Randomisation:		
Sequence generation	8a	Method used to generate the random allocation sequence
	8b	Type of randomisation; details of any restriction (such as blocking and block size)
Allocation concealment mechanism	9	Mechanism used to implement the random allocation sequence (such as sequentially numbered containers), describing any steps taken to conceal the sequence until interventions were assigned
Implementation	10	Who generated the random allocation sequence, who enrolled participants, and who assigned participants to interventions
Blinding	11a	If done, who was blinded after assignment to interventions (for example, participants, care providers, those assessing outcomes) and how
	11b	If relevant, description of the similarity of interventions
Statistical methods	12a	Statistical methods used to compare groups for primary and secondary outcomes
	12b	Methods for additional analyses, such as subgroup analyses and adjusted analyses
Results		
Participant flow (a diagram is strongly recommended)	13a	For each group, the numbers of participants who were randomly assigned, received intended treatment, and were analysed for the primary outcome
	13b	For each group, losses and exclusions after randomisation, together with reasons
Recruitment	14a	Dates defining the periods of recruitment and follow-up

	14b	Why the trial ended or was stopped
Baseline data	15	A table showing baseline demographic and clinical characteristics for each group
Numbers analysed	16	For each group, number of participants (denominator) included in each analysis and whether the analysis was by original assigned groups
Outcomes and estimation	17a	For each primary and secondary outcome, results for each group, and the estimated effect size and its precision (such as 95% confidence interval)
	17b	For binary outcomes, presentation of both absolute and relative effect sizes is recommended
Ancillary analyses	18	Results of any other analyses performed, including subgroup analyses and adjusted analyses, distinguishing pre-specified from exploratory
Harms	19	All important harms or unintended effects in each group (for specific guidance see CONSORT for harms)
Discussion		
Limitations	20	Trial limitations, addressing sources of potential bias, imprecision, and, if relevant, multiplicity of analyses
Generalisability	21	Generalisability (external validity, applicability) of the trial findings
Interpretation	22	Interpretation consistent with results, balancing benefits and harms, and considering other relevant evidence
Other information		
Registration	23	Registration number and name of trial registry
Protocol	24	Where the full trial protocol can be accessed, if available
Funding	25	Sources of funding and other support (such as supply of drugs), role of funders

CONSORT flowchart (Fig. 15.1)

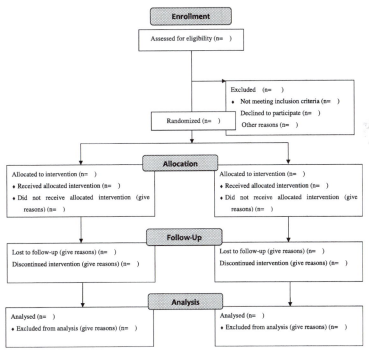

FIGURE 15.1   CONSORT 2010 flowchart.

STROBE statement (Table 15.5)

TABLE 15.5 Checklist for observational studies.

	No.	recommendation
Title and abstract	1	(a) Identify the study design in the title or abstract using a commonly used term
		(b) For the abstract, write a meaningful and balanced summary of what was done in the study and what was found out
introduction		
Background/ Rational	2nd	Explain the scientific background and the rationale for the study presented
Objectives	3rd	State all specific objectives including the (pre-defined) hypotheses
Methods		
Study design	4th	Describe the most important elements of the study design as early as possible in the article
frame	5	Describe the framework (setting) and location of the study and provide relevant time information, including the periods of recruitment, exposure, follow-up and data collection
Study participants	6	(a) Cohort study - indicate the inclusion criteria, the origin of the participants and the methods of their selection; describe the methods of follow-up case control study - specify the inclusion criteria and the origin of the cases and controls, and the methods by which the cases were collected and controls selected. Provide a rationale for the selection of cases and controls. Cross-sectional study - specify the inclusion criteria, the origin of the participants and the methods of their selection
		(b) Cohort study - For studies that use matching, specify the matching criteria and the number of exposed and unexposed participants in the case control study - For studies that use matching, enter the matching criteria and the number of Controls per case
variables	7	Clearly define all targets, exposures, predictors, possible confounders and effect modifiers; if necessary, enter diagnostic criteria
Data sources / Measurement methods	8th*	Specify the data sources for each important variable in the study and explain the assessment and measurement methods used. Describe the comparability of the measurement methods if there is more than one group
Bias	9	Describe what has been done to address possible causes of bias
Study size	10th	Explain how the study size was determined
Quantitative variables	11	Explain how quantitative variables were dealt with in the evaluations. If necessary, describe how categories (groupings) were formed and why
Statistical methods	12th	(a) Describe all statistical methods, including those used to control confounding
		(b) Describe procedures used to examine subgroups and interactions
		(c) Explain how missing data was handled
		(d) Cohort study - If necessary, explain how the problem of early withdrawal from the study ("loss to follow-up") was dealt with - If necessary, describe the evaluation methods that take into account the selected sampling strategy
		(e) Describe sensitivity analyzes
Results		
Attendees	13 *	(a) Enter the number of participants during each study phase, e.g. For example, the number of participants who were potentially eligible, who were screened for eligibility, who were confirmed to be eligible, who actually participated in the study, whose follow-up was completed, and whose data were evaluated
		(b) State the reasons for not participating in each study phase
		(c) Consider representation in a flow chart
Descriptive data	14 *	(a) Describe the characteristics of the study participants (e.g. demographic, clinical and social characteristics) as well as exposures and possible confounders
		(b) Enter the number of participants with missing data for each variable
		(c) Cohort study - summarize the follow-up time (e.g. mean and total period)
Result data	15 *	Cohort study - report on the number of target events or statistical measures (e.g. mean and standard deviation) over time Case control study - report on the number of participants in each exposure category or statistical measures of exposure (e.g. mean and standard deviation) Cross-sectional study - Report the number of target events or statistical measures (e.g. mean and standard deviation)
Main results	16	(a) State the unadjusted estimates and, if necessary, also the estimates in which adjustments were made for the confounders and their precision (e.g. 95% confidence interval); make it clear which confounder was adjusted and why it was taken into account
		(b) If continuous variables have been categorized, provide the upper and lower limits of each category
		(c) If relevant, consider expressing relative risk estimates as absolute risks for meaningful periods
Further evaluations	17th	Report on other evaluations made, e.g. B. Analysis of subgroups and interactions (interactions) as well as sensitivity analysis discussion
Main results	18th	Summarize the most important results regarding the study goals
limitations	19th	Discuss the limitations of the study, taking into account the reasons for possible bias or imprecision. Discuss the direction and extent of each possible bias
interpretation	20th	Cautiously interpret the results, taking into account the goals and limitations of the study, the multiplicity of the analyzes, the results of other studies, and other relevant evidence
Portability	21	Discuss the portability (external validity) of the study results. Additional information
financing	22	Indicate how this study was funded and explain the role of donors. If necessary, provide this information for the original study on which this article is based

* Provide this information separately for cases and controls in case control studies, and where appropriate for exposed and non-exposed groups in cohort and cross-sectional studies.
Note : Each item on the checklist is discussed in an accompanying article (Explanation and Elaboration), which discusses methodological backgrounds and presents published examples of transparent reporting. The STROBE checklist is best used with this article (freely available on the following websites: PLoS Medicine http://www.plosmedicine.org, Annals of Internal Medicine http://www.annals.org and Epidemiology http: / /www.epidem.com). Additional versions of the checklist specific to cohort, case control or cross-sectional studies are available on the STROBE website (http://www.strobe-statement.org) in English.

SIGN 50 for systematic review and meta analysis (Table 15.6)

TABLE 15.6 SIGN 50 checklist for systematic review and meta analysis.

SIGN	Methodology Checklist 1: Systematic Reviews and Meta-analyzes		
Study identification (*Include author, title, year of publication, journal title, pages*)			
Guideline topic:		Key question no:	
Before completing this checklist, consider: Is the paper a systematic review or meta-analysis? IF NO REJECT (give reason below). IF YES CONTINUE. Is the paper relevant to key question? Analysis using PICO (Patient or Population Intervention Comparison Outcome). IF NO REJECT (give reason below). IF YES complete the checklist.			
Reason for rejection: 1. Paper not a systematic review / meta-analysis □ 2. Paper not relevant to key question □ 3. Other reason □ (please specify):			
Checklist completed by:			
Section 1: Internal validity			
In a well conducted systematic review		In this study this criterion is ::	
1.1	The study addresses an appropriate and clearly focused question.	Well covered Adequately addressed Poorly addressed	Not addressed Not reported Not applicable
1.2	A description of the methodology used is included.	Well covered Adequately addressed Poorly addressed	Not addressed Not reported Not applicable
1.3	*The literature search is sufficiently rigorous to identify all the relevant studies.*	Well covered Adequately addressed Poorly addressed	Not addressed Not reported Not applicable
1.4	Study quality is assessed and taken into account.	Well covered Adequately addressed Poorly addressed	Not addressed Not reported Not applicable
1.5	There are enough similarities between the studies selected to make combining them reasonable.	Well covered Adequately addressed Poorly addressed	Not addressed Not reported Not applicable
Section 2: OVERALL ASSESSMENT OF THE			
2.1	*How well was the study done to minimize bias?* Code ++, +, or –		
2.2	Notes. Summarise the authors conclusions. Add any comments on your own assessment of the study, and the extent to which it answers your question.		

SIGN 50 for randomized controlled trials (Table 15.7)

TABLE 15.7 SIGN 50 checklist for systematic review and meta analysis.

SIGN	Methodology Checklist 2: Randomized Controlled Trials		
Study identification (Include *author, title, year of publication, journal title, pages*)			
Guideline topic:		Key question no:	
Checklist completed by:			
Section 1: Internal validity			
In a well conducted RCT study… ..		**In this study this criterion is**	
1.1	The study addresses an appropriate and clearly focused question.	Well covered	Not addressed
		Adequately addressed	Not reported
		Poorly addressed	Not applicable
1.2	The assignment of subjects to treatment groups is randomized	Well covered	Not addressed
		Adequately addressed	Not reported
		Poorly addressed	Not applicable
1.3	An adequate concealment method is used	Well covered	Not addressed
		Adequately addressed	Not reported
		Poorly addressed	Not applicable
1.4	Subjects and investigators are kept 'blind' about treatment allocation	Well covered	Not addressed
		Adequately addressed	Not reported
		Poorly addressed	Not applicable
1.5	The treatment and control groups are similar at the start of the trial	Well covered	Not addressed
		Adequately addressed	Not reported
		Poorly addressed	Not applicable
1.6	The only difference between groups is the treatment under investigation	Well covered	Not addressed
		Adequately addressed	Not reported
		Poorly addressed	Not applicable
1.7	All relevant outcomes are measured in a standard, valid and reliable way	Well covered	Not addressed
		Adequately addressed	Not reported
		Poorly addressed	Not applicable
1.8	What percentage of the individuals or clusters recruited into each treatment arm of the study dropped out before the study was completed?		
1.9	All the subjects are analyzed in the groups to which they were randomly allocated (often referred to as intention to treat analysis)	Well covered	Not addressed
		Adequately addressed	Not reported
		Poorly addressed	Not applicable
1.10	Where the study is carried out at more than one site, results are comparable for all sites	Well covered	Not addressed
		Adequately addressed	Not reported
		Poorly addressed	Not applicable

Section 2: OVERALL ASSESSMENT OF THE STUDY		
2.1	How well was the study done to minimize bias? Code ++, +, or −	
2.2	If coded as +, or −□what is the likely direction in which bias might affect the study results?	
2.3	Taking into account clinical considerations, your evaluation of the methodology used, and the statistical power of the study, are you certain that the overall effect is due to the study intervention?	
2.4	Are the results of this study directly applicable to the patient group targeted by this guideline?	
Section 3: DESCRIPTION OF THE STUDY (The following information is required to complete evidence tables facilitating cross-study comparisons. Please complete all sections for which information is available). PLEASE PRINT CLEARLY		
3.1	How many patients are included in this study? *Please indicate number in each arm of the study, at the time the study began.*	
3.2	What are the main characteristics of the patient population? *Include all relevant characteristics - eg age, sex, ethnic origin, comorbidity, disease status, community / hospital based*	
3.3	What intervention (treatment, procedure) is being investigated in this study? *List all interventions covered by the study.*	
3.4	What comparisons are made in the study? *Are comparisons made between treatments, or between treatment and placebo / no treatment?*	
3.5	How long are patients followed-up in the study? *Length of time patients are followed from beginning participation in the study. Note specified end points used to decide end of follow-up (eg death, complete cure). Note if follow-up period is shorter than originally planned.*	
3.6	What outcome measure (s) are used in the study? *List all outcomes that are used to assess effectiveness of the interventions used.*	
3.7	What size of effect is identified in the study? *List all measures of effect in the units used in the study - eg absolute or relative risk, NNT, etc. Include p values and any confidence intervals that are provided.*	
3.8	How was this study funded? *List all sources of funding quoted in the article, whether Government, voluntary sector, or industry.*	
3.9	Does this study help to answer your key question? *Summarise the main conclusions of the study and indicate how it relates to the key question.*	

SIGN 50 for cohort study (Table 15.8)

TABLE 15.8 SIGN 50 for cohort study.

	Methodology Checklist 3: Cohort studies		
SIGN			
	Study identification (Include *author, title, year of publication, journal title, pages*)		
Guideline topic:		Key question no:	
Before completing this checklist, consider: Is the paper really a cohort study? If in doubt, check the study design algorithm available from SIGN and make sure you have the correct checklist. Is the paper relevant to key question? Analysis using PICO (Patient or Population Intervention Comparison Outcome). IF NO REJECT (give reason below). IF YES complete the checklist ..			
Reason for rejection: 1. Paper not relevant to key question □ 2. Other reason □ (please specify):			
Checklist completed by:			
Section 1: Internal validity			
In a well conducted cohort study:		In this study the criterion is:	
1.1	The study addresses an appropriate and clearly focused question.	Well covered Adequately addressed Poorly addressed	Not addressed Not reported Not applicable
Selection of subjects			
1.2	The two groups being studied are selected from source populations that are comparable in all respects other than the factor under investigation.	Well covered Adequately addressed Poorly addressed	Not addressed Not reported Not applicable
1.3	The study indicates how many of the people asked to take part did so, in each of the groups being studied.	Well covered Adequately addressed Poorly addressed	Not addressed Not reported Not applicable
1.4	The likelihood that some eligible subjects might have the outcome at the time of enrollment is assessed and taken into account in the analysis.	Well covered Adequately addressed Poorly addressed	Not addressed Not reported Not applicable
1.5	What percentage of individuals or clusters recruited into each arm of the study dropped out before the study was completed.		
1.6	Comparison is made between full participants and those lost to follow up, by exposure status.	Well covered Adequately addressed Poorly addressed	Not addressed Not reported Not applicable
ASSESSMENT			
1.7	The outcomes are clearly defined.	Well covered Adequately addressed Poorly addressed	Not addressed Not reported Not applicable
1.8	The assessment of outcome is made blind to exposure status.	Well covered Adequately addressed Poorly addressed	Not addressed Not reported Not applicable
1.9	Where blinding was not possible, there is some recognition that knowledge of exposure status could have influenced the assessment of outcome.	Well covered Adequately addressed Poorly addressed	Not addressed Not reported Not applicable
1.10	The measure of assessment of exposure is reliable.	Well covered Adequately addressed Poorly addressed	Not addressed Not reported Not applicable
1.11	Evidence from other sources is used to demonstrate that the method of outcome assessment is valid and reliable.	Well covered Adequately addressed Poorly addressed	Not addressed Not reported Not applicable
1.12	Exposure level or prognostic factor is assessed more than once.	Well covered Adequately addressed Poorly addressed	Not addressed Not reported Not applicable
CONFOUNDING			
1.13	The main potential confounders are identified and taken into account in the design and analysis.	Well covered Adequately addressed Poorly addressed	Not addressed Not reported Not a pplicable
STATISTICAL ANALYSIS			
1.14	Have confidence intervals been provided?		
Section 2: OVERALL ASSESSMENT OF THE STUDY			
2.1	How well was the study done to minimize the risk of bias or confounding, and to establish a causal relationship between exposure and effect? *Code ++, +, or −*		
2.2	Taking into account clinical considerations, your evaluation of the methodology used, and the statistical power of the study, are you certain that the overall effect is due to the study intervention?		
2.3	Are the results of this study directly applicable to the patient group targeted in this guideline?		

2.4	Notes. Summarise the authors conclusions. Add any comments on your own assessment of the study, and the extent to which it answers your question.	

The following section is provided for non-SIGN users of this checklist and is being developed to conform to the standards set by the Guidelines International Network Evidence Tables Working Group.
Members of SIGN guideline groups do not need to complete this section.

Section 3: description OF THE STUDY
PLEASE PRINT CLEARLY

3.1	*Do we know who the study was funded by?*	□ Academic Institution □ Healthcare Industry □ Government □ NGO □ Public funds □ Other
3.2	*How many centers are patients recruited from?*	
3.3	*From which countries are patients selected? (Select all those involved. Note additional countries after "Other")*	□ Scotland □ UK □ USA □ Canada □ Australia □ New Zealand □ France □ Germany □ Italy □ Netherlands □ Scandinavia □ Spain □ Other:
3.4	*What is the social setting (ie type of environment in which they live) of patients in the study?*	□ Urban □ Rural □ Mixed
3.5	*What criteria are used to decide who should be INCLUDED in the study?*	
3.6	*What criteria are used to decide who should be EXCLUDED from the study?*	
3.7	*What intervention or risk factor is investigated in the study? (Include dosage where appropriate)*	
3.8	*What comparisons are made in the study (ie what alternative treatments are used to compare the intervention / exposure with). Include dosage where appropriate.*	
3.9	*What methods were used to randomize patients, blind patients or investigators, and to conceal the randomization process from investigators?*	
3.10	*How long did the active phase of the study last?*	
3.11	*How long were patients followed-up for, during and after the study?*	
3.12	*List the key characteristics of the patient population. Note if there are any significant differences between different arms of the trial.*	

3.13	*Record the basic data for each arm of the study. If there are more than four arms, note data for subsequent arms at the bottom of the page.*			
	Arm 1: Treatment: Sample size: No. analyzed With outcome: Without outcome:	Arm 2: Treatment: Sample size: No. analyzed With outcome: Without outcome> Primary outcome?	Arm 3: Treatment: Sample size: No. analyzed With outcome: Without outcome> Primary outcome?	Arm 4: Treatment: Sample size: No. analyzed With outcome: Without outcome Primary outcome?

3.14	*Record the basic data for each IMPORTANT outcome in the study. If there are more than four, not data for additional outcomes at the bottom of the page.*			
	Outcome 1: Value: Measure: P value Upper CI Lower CI Primary outcome?	Outcome 2: Value: Measure: P value Upper CI Lower CI Primary outcome?	Outcome 3: Value: Measure: P value Upper CI Lower CI Primary outcome?	Outcome 4: Value: Measure: P value Upper CI Lower CI Primary outcome?

3.15	Notes. Summarise the authors conclusions. Add any comments on your own assessment of the study, and the extent to which it answers your question. *(Much of this is likely to be contributed by GDG members).*	

SIGN 50 for case control study (Table 15.9)

TABLE 15.9 SIGN 50 for case control study.

SIGN	Methodology Checklist 4: Case-control studies		
	Study identification (Include *author, title, year of publication, journal title, pages*)		
Guideline topic:		Key question no:	
Before completing this checklist, consider: Is the paper really a case-control study? If in doubt, check the study design algorithm available from SIGN and make sure you have the correct checklist. Is the paper relevant to key question? Analysis using PICO (Patient or Population Intervention Comparison Outcome). IF NO REJECT (give reason below). IF YES complete the checklist.			
Reason for rejection: Reason for rejection: 1. Paper not relevant to key question □ 2. Other reason □ (please specify):			
Checklist completed by:			
Section 1: Internal validity			
In an well conducted case control study:		In this study the criterion is:	
1.1	The study addresses an appropriate and clearly focused question	Well covered Adequately addressed Poorly addressed	Not addressed Not reported Not applicable
Selection of subjects			
1.2	The cases and controls are taken from comparable populations	Well covered Adequately addressed Poorly addressed	Not addressed Not reported Not applicable
1.3	The same exclusion criteria are used for both cases and controls	Well covered Adequately addressed Poorly addressed	Not addressed Not reported Not applicable
1.4	What percentage of each group (cases and controls) participated in the study?	Cases: Controls:	
1.5	Comparison is made between participants and non-participants to establish their similarities or differences	Well covered Adequately addressed Poorly addressed	Not addressed Not reported Not applicable
1.6	Cases are clearly defined and differentiated from controls	Well covered Adequately addressed Poorly addressed	Not addressed Not reported Not applicable
1.7	It is clearly established that controls are non-cases	Well covered Adequately addressed Poorly addressed	Not addressed Not reported Not applicable
ASSESSMENT			
1.8	Measures will have been taken to prevent knowledge of primary exposure influencing case ascertainment	Well covered Adequately addressed Poorly addressed	Not addressed Not reported Not applicable
1.9	Exposure status is measured in a standard, valid and reliable way	Well covered Adequately addressed Poorly addressed	Not addressed Not reported Not applicable
CONFOUNDING			
1.10	The main potential confounders are identified and taken into account in the design and analysis	Well covered Adequately addressed Poorly addressed	Not addressed Not reported Not applicable
STATISTICAL ANALYSIS			
1.11	Confidence intervals are provided		
Section 2: OVERALL ASSESSMENT OF THE STUDY			
2.1	How well was the study done to minimize the risk of bias or confounding? Code ++, +, or −		
2.2	Taking into account clinical considerations, your evaluation of the methodology used, and the statistical power of the study, are you certain that the overall effect is due to the study intervention?		
2.3	Are the results of this study directly applicable to the patient group targeted by this guideline?		
2.4	Notes. Summarise the authors conclusions. Add any comments on your own assessment of the study, and the extent to which it answers your question.		
The following section is provided for non-SIGN users of this checklist and is being developed to conform to the standards set by the Guidelines International Network Evidence Tables Working Group. *Members of SIGN guideline groups do not need to complete this section.*			
Section 3: description OF THE STUDY PLEASE PRINT CLEARLY			
3.1	*Do we know who the study was funded by?*	□ Academic Institution □ Healthcare Industry □ Government □ NGO □ Public funds □ Other	
3.2	*How many centers are patients recruited from?*		
3.3	*From which countries are patients selected? (Select all those involved. Note additional countries after " Other ")*	□ Scotland □ UK □ USA □ Canada □ Australia □ New Zealand □ France □ Germany □ Italy □ Netherlands □ Scandinavia □ Spain □ Other:	
3.4	*What is the social setting (ie type of environment in which they live) of patients in the study?*	□ Urban □ Rural □ Mixed	
3.5	*What criteria are used to decide who should be cases?*		
3.6	What criteria are used to decide who should be controls?		
3.7	*What exposure or risk factor is investigated in the study? (Include dosage where appropriate)*		
3.8	*How long were patients followed-up for?*		
3.9	*List the key characteristics of the patient population. Note if there are any significant differences between different arms of the trial.*		
3.10	*Record the basic data for each arm of the study. If there are more than four arms, note data for subsequent arms at the bottom of the page.*		
	Cases: Exposure: Sample size: No. analyzed With outcome: Without outcome:	Cases: Exposure: Sample size: No. analyzed With outcome: Without outcome:	
3.11	Notes. Summarise the authors conclusions. Add any comments on your own assessment of the study, and the extent to which it answers your question. *(Much of this is likely to be contributed by GDG members).*		

Index

Note: Page numbers followed by "*f*" and "*t*" refer to figures and tables, respectively.

Printed in the United States
by Baker & Taylor Publisher Services